Pāgalāmi: Ethnopsychiatric Knowledge in Bengal

Deborah P. Bhattacharyya

Foreign and Comparative Studies/South Asian Series, No. 11
Maxwell School of Citizenship and Public Affairs
Syracuse University
1986

Portions of this book originally appeared in
Contributions to Asian Studies 18 (1984)
and *Social Science and Medicine* XVII (1983),
as articles entitled
"Desire in Bengali Ethnopsychology"
and "Psychiatric Pluralism in Bengal, India,"
respectively.
REPRINTED WITH PERMISSION.

Library of Congress Cataloging in Publication Data
Bhattacharyya, Deborah P., 1943-
Pagalami : ethnopsychiatric knowledge in Bengal.

(Foreign and comparative studies. South Asian series ; no. 11)
Bibliography: p.
Includes indew.
1. Psychiatry--India--Bengal. 2. Mental illness--India--Bengal. 3. Social psychiatry--India--Bengal.
I. Title. II. Series.
RC451.I6B26 1986 616.89'00954'14 86-8639
ISBN 0-915984-89-X

CONTENTS

LIST OF TABLES

LIST OF FIGURES

ACKNOWLEDGMENTS

Fieldwork for this research was conducted in 1975-76 with support from the Social Science Research Council - American Council of Learned Societies. A return visit during the summer of 1982 was made possible through a faculty development grant from DePauw University.

My thanks and appreciation go to the members of my dissertation committee: Whitney Pope, Bill Corsaro, Larry Hazelrigg, Ivan Karp, and Ralph Nicholas. Dr. Charles Leslie has been very supportive of my work. I also want to acknowledge the special help of Tarun Mitra, Dr. P.K. Bhowmick, Dr. Ajita Chakraborty, Dr. Suhas Chatterjee, Shipra Chatterjee, and Aditi Nath Sarkar. The psychiatric community, specialists and clients, extended great hospitality to me in Calcutta, for which I am very appreciative. Mary Beth Ritter has been an understanding, patient, but most importantly, a totally competent editor.

My thanks and love to all those friends and family who gave their support and encouragement and sustained me through the inevitable troughs of doing research. My daughers Karabi and Ketaki have probably not made this research any easier, but they have certainly made my efforts more worthwhile.

INTRODUCTION

Studying the Psychiatric Domain in Bengal

Calcutta, the major city of the state of West Bengal in eastern India, first impressed me as being incredibly chaotic. It is extremely crowded, with winding alleys leading into narrow lanes which, in turn, run into major roads. Traffic is a nightmare, with trams, buses, taxis, man-pulled carts, rickshaws and pedestrians all vying for what little space there is. Being a passenger in a swerving car seems bad enough, but being a pedestrian is an exercise in total frustration. The pathways are often jammed with vendors' makeshift stands, leaving only a very narrow passage barely sufficient for two people walking in opposite directions. As I found myself bumped and pushed at every step of the way, I condemned Bengalis for their lack of concern with order.

Several months later, however, I could walk for blocks without bumping into a single person. What was the cause of this miraculous change? Quite simply, I had identified a basic social norm of Bengali pedestrians: stay on the left side of the pathway. Part of India's British heritage was the adoption of the British traffic pattern, which is also used by pedestrian traffic. As an American, I had been blithely walking on the right -- smack into the oncoming flow from the opposite direction. But once I had learned the appropriate cultural rule, the apparent chaos vanished and the underlying order was suddenly so clear that I wondered how I could ever have missed it.

This experience of order emerging out of perceptual chaos was repeated in my research on mental illness in Bengal. At first, I was mentally bumped and pushed by the disjointed bits and pieces of data I was collecting. What I had to do as an analyst was to put together these bits and pieces into an organized and meaningful set. I had to locate the social norms or cultural rules underlying the behavioral patterns I was observing. In studying mental illness in Bengal, I had to identify the conceptual categories that Bengalis themselves use. As long as I relied on my own expectations and ideas about mental illness, I would, in effect, keep "bumping into" and never understanding the world as Bengalis know it.

Sociology of Knowledge

In focusing on Bengali conceptions of mental illness, I am adopting a phenomenological approach. For Schutz (1970), the task of sociology is an investigation of the commonsense knowledge of the world of everyday life. Applying this approach to my research means that I have studied the social knowledge that Bengalis have about mental illness. In anthropology, such an approach is often termed an "emic" orientation (Pike, 1954) or "ethnoscience" (Sturtevant, 1964), because it investigates the conceptual frameworks that are meaningful to those being studied. Ethnopsychiatry, then, is the study of indigenous conceptions of psychiatric disorder.

My approach to sociology of knowledge makes three assumptions about human knowledge. First, reality as experienced by human beings is a constructed phenomenon. Like Schutz, I reject a naive realism which views the reality of the world as passively received. Rather than merely reflecting an independent external reality, human knowledge is one of the means by which a reality is established. Second, human knowledge is a process that involves social activity and therefore is rooted in the dynamics of the social order which generates it. Similarly, the social order itself is conceived as the concrete processes of specific individuals acting in particular social settings. Third, in spite of the social nature of knowledge, both in terms of its emergence and its consequences, a sociological determinism with regards to knowledge is unacceptable. The active, creative potential of individuals, albeit situated in and therefore affected by a particular socio-cultural-physical environment, is clearly recognized.

Since both knowledge and the social order to which it pertains are emergent products of ongoing social activity, the reification of society or of knowledge is carefully avoided. Knowledge is always in the knowing of it (i.e., social activity), and social activity always implies a cognitive function inherent in it. To talk of knowledge without ultimate reference to the social existential conditions in which it is situated is to be involved in what Marx might call alienated thought and the ideological practice of science (see Smith, 1974). To talk of social phenomena without reference to the knowledge and meaning they entail is to be involved in what the phenomenologists have decried as the objectivication of man (Giorgi, 1970; Bittner, 1973). Knowledge and social activity mutually imply each other.[1]

The primary goal of this research is an analysis of the psychiatric domain through an analysis of the conceptual meanings inherent in the Bengali term pāgalāmi, variously translated as mental illness, madness, or insanity.[2] The research examines the sociocultural meanings of pāgalāmi by identifying the ethnopsychiatric theories which make pāgalāmi a meaningful concept to Bengali actors. It is important, however, to distinguish between pāgalāmi as concept and pāgalāmi as phenomenon. While it is the concept of pāgalāmi which is the subject of this book, for Bengalis pāgalāmi is not merely a concept but a real and objectively existing phenomenon. From this point of view, one of the key characteristics of the concept is that it accords its referent an ontological status as a phenomenon which exists in the real world. This characteristic of knowledge can be referred to as the reflexivity of knowledge: Knowledge produces the very phenomenon to which it refers. The use of the concept pāgalāmi in the situated context of everyday social action asserts the ontological status of its referent, and thereby produces the phenomenon pāgalāmi. The concept of pāgalāmi affirms the existence of the phenomenon pāgalāmi as a thing or entity, independent from the thought of the actors themselves. It is in this regard that knowledge can be seen as creating the phenomenal world for the actors.

Thus, an investigation of the psychiatric domain in Bengal is ultimately an investigation of the processes by which pāgalāmi becomes constituted as an observable objective phenomenon for the actors themselves. It is, in this sense, an investigation of the production and accomplishment of pāgalāmi among Bengalis. Furthermore, an analysis of the concept of pāgalāmi must entail an inquiry into the theories that the actors use in order to produce pāgalāmi as phenomenon. Pāgalāmi is possible as a phenomenon because Bengalis have and use theories which provide for its existence. Conversely, pāgalāmi is not possible among Americans because they do not share the relevant theories of the world.

This point can be illustrated by using the example of mental illness as a phenomenon (i.e., rather than as a concept). Mental illness, as a disease of the mind, is possible only to the extent that individuals use theories which identify the mind as the kind of entity that can become diseased. Szasz's critique of mental illness (1970, 1974) is essentially an argument declaring such theories and the medical model of mind invalid. Because he believes that mind cannot be appropriately linked to the phenomenon of disease, Szasz denies the possibility of mental illness and concludes that it is a "myth." Similarly, mental illness, as a disease of the mind, requires theories which establish mind as a phenomenon differentiated from other phenomena, such as body. Therefore, mental illness -- again as a disease of the mind -- is not possible as a differentiated experiential phenomenon among the inhabitants of the Chiapas highlands in Mexico because of the unity they perceive between mind and body (Manning and Fabrega, 1973).

Thus, an adequate analysis of a concept, such as pāgalāmi, must elaborate the theories that social actors use in order to produce the phenomenon referred to by the concept.[3] To describe the theorizing relevant to the production of pāgalāmi and thereby to describe the psychiatric domain in Bengal, I have differentiated theorizing about pāgalāmi into two separate categories: theories which establish the internal structure of the psychiatric domain, and theories which locate the psychiatric domain within the broader sociocultural context of Bengal. Some of the theories in the first category establish boundaries around that domain by differentiating pāgalāmi from other phenomena. These are the theories that Bengalis invoke in order to perceive and identify someone as pāgala [the adjective derived from the noun pāgalāmi]. Other theories about the internal structure of the psychiatric domain make distinctions which differentiate some pāgalāmi as being different from other pāgalāmi. The second category, theorizing which contextualizes the psychiatric domain within Bengali culture, includes theories which specify the nature of a person or event implied through the label pāgalāmi. In this way, such theories identify pāgalāmi as an instance of a broader phenomenon.

Methodology and Data Collection

The theoretical orientation discussed above argues that knowledge must be analyzed as the emergent product of social activity. Knowledge is constituted by virtue of practices which depend for their very coherence and meaningfulness upon the knowledge they produce. Since knowledge ultimately refers to situated social activity and practices, research must be identified in terms of specific social activity. This study involved data collection and analysis of two types of social behavior: treatment-seeking behavior and the performative use of language.

One major category of social activity investigated is that surrounding the provision of treatment for those identified as pāgala. The provision of psychiatric treatment in Bengal has been institutionalized to a large degree, and thus it is possible to identify the social institutions which provide such treatment. These institutions are based upon a particular set of role relationships: those involving a psychiatric specialist (who provides treatment), a psychiatric client (who seeks treatment), and a psychiatric patient (who receives treatment). Analysis of this set of role relationships is one of the main strategies used to organize the presentation of the research findings.

A second major category of social activity examined is verbal behavior, i.e., interview data. Several scholars of language have noted that the social use of language extends beyond the communication of cognitive content and includes various social actions. Talk not only tells of something, but also enables the speaker to perform certain activities. Austin (1962) has called such talk "performatives," and others have argued that all speech can be analyzed in terms of "the actions that are being performed by speakers through their utterances" (Labov and Fanshel 1977:58). Accordingly, the interviews I conducted are analyzed in terms of the social activity they enable the respondent to perform. For example, judgments about who is or is not pāgala constitute a procedure for establishing boundaries around the psychiatric domain. Verbal behavior "about" pāgalāmi is a social activity which constructs pāgalāmi as a differentiated and experiential phenomenon, and is thus a major source of data for this study.

The research for this book was conducted in 1975-76 among Bengali-language speakers living in and around Calcutta. Thus, even though "Bengal" and hence the adjective "Bengali" apply to both the state of West Bengal in eastern India and the nation of Bangladesh, this research focuses on the former. The present population of West Bengal, comprising both indigenous inhabitants and immigrants from Bangladesh, is predominately Hindu, with a sizable Muslim minority. The data reported, however, were collected almost exclusively from Hindu respondents. Bengali Hindus are patrilineal, view the patrilocal joint families as the cultural ideal, and, like other Hindus in India, share the Sanskritic tradition and a caste hierarchy.

Though the data collected in the various settings were quite varied, three major kinds of data emerged, a summary of which is presented in Table 1. The first of these includes contacts with relatives of outpatients. At Western-style allopathic clinics in Bhowanipore and Ranaghat, as well as at the curing temples, I interviewed persons who brought relatives for outpatient psychiatric treatment. The main focus of these unstructured interviews was the patient's case history and the relative's perception of important symptoms, etiological factors, possible diagnosis, and appropriate treatment. These interviews included such questions as: What symptoms has the patient exhibited which made you decide to seek treatment? What do you think is the matter with the patient? Do others have different ideas about what the problem is? Why do you think the patient became ill? What things do you think could have caused the present illness? How did you decide to bring the patient here? What other treatment has the patient already received? Are you considering any other treatment?

The second category of data involved interviews with mental health practitioners. These include allopathic psychiatrists, Ayurvedic doctors, folk healers, and the priests at the curing temples. In these interviews,

TABLE 1

Data Sources

Category of Data	
I. Patients and Their Relatives	
A. Bhowanipore - Observe Psychiatric Interviews	120
B. Bhowanipore - Interviews with Relatives	44
C. Ranaghat - Interviews with Relatives	12
D. Curing Temples - Interviews with Relatives	4
II. Mental Health Professionals	
A. Psychiatrists and Psychoanalysts	30
B. Ayurvedic Practitioners	7
C. Folk Healers	6
D. Priests at Curing Temples	5
III. Star Questionnaires	
A. Psychiatrists and Psychoanalysts	30
B. Urban Middle Class (Calcutta)	30
C. Semi-rural, Lower Middle Class (Dishergarh)	30
D. All-Bengal Women's Union Home for Women	30

I asked the practitioners about their particular theoretical orientation to mental illness as well as their clinical experiences with mental illness in Bengal.

Finally, structured questionnaires were administered to four samples of 30 persons each: allopathic psychiatrists and psychoanalysts; urban middle-class respondents; semi-rural lower-middle-class respondents from the village of Dishergarh, and residents of the All Bengal Women's Union Home for Women, a home for girls and young women abandoned by their families. The questionnaire (see Appendix A) was a Bengali translation of the format by Star (see Joint Commission on Mental Illness and Health, 1961), with six different "cases," each portraying one of the Western psychiatric diagnostic categories of mental illness. The respondents were then asked whether those described are abnormal, whether they are mentally ill, and what, if anything, should be done.

One of the strengths of my research is the diversity of the populations surveyed. As noted above, the Bengalis I interviewed can be divided into three main groups relative to their position in the psychiatric domain: those concerned with providing treatment, those concerned with obtaining treatment for the patient, and Bengalis who were peripheral to the psychiatric domain. Similarly, my research familiarized me with a number of distinctive settings within the psychiatric domain. I had extensive contact with Western psychiatric medicine and considerable contact with both Ayurveda (traditional, Sanskritic medicine) and folk medicine (that practiced by an ōjhā). Relatives were usually contacted at Western-style clinics, but they provided a great deal of data on other medical systems. This diversity enables a composite view of the psychiatric domain which would have been impossible if data had been collected from only one or two of these groups.

While those interviewed were almost exclusively Hindu, the population did represent considerable socioeconomic heterogeneity. At one end of the social hierarchy are the allopathic psychiatrists and some of the other professionals who were part of the sample I have designated as urban middle class. The majority of the middle-class males, however, were less educated and had lower-level professional, governmental, or business occupations. Their orientation to traditional Bengali culture varied, but in general they felt rooted in that tradition while at the same time striving to be "modern." Women of this class were less educated, generally unemployed, and tended to be more traditional in outlook. Persons of this status are not highly represented (less than 15 percent) among the samples of patients' relatives because they prefer private psychiatrists to the clinics where I conducted interviews.

Lower-middle-class persons were the dominant group at Bhowanipore and in the Dishergarh sample. Dishergarh is a small village near Asansol, and those interviewed were from families of the lower-level clerical employees of the mining corporation. At Bhowanipore, approximately one-third of the patients came from urban Calcutta families whose primary wage earners held similar white-collar clerical positions in business or government service.

The lower socioeconomic classes, both urban and rural, were not highly represented in my samples. Still, they did bring patients to Bhowanipore, to Ranaghat and to the curing temples. About 20 percent of the Bhowanipore patients came from a rural background (primarily small cultivators or tenant farmers), while slightly less than a third came from families with non-white-collar wage earners. The residents of the All Bengal Women's Union

Home came primarily from rural and lower-class backgrounds, and some of them had maintained contact with their kin groups. However, they were educated at the Home and also trained in semi-skilled occupations such as tailoring, characteristics which are not typical for women of their class position in Bengali society. Many of them seemed to aspire to lower-middle-class status, but their origins and present situation were hindrances in arranging the kind of marriage needed to validate that status. In attitude as well, I suspect they were suspended between the orientations of their natal families and those of the upper middle-class women who ran the Home.[4]

Overview

In summary, this book explores the relationship between knowledge and social behavior within the psychiatric domain in Bengal. It analyzes social activity within that domain and the knowledge which exists as the emergent social product of that activity. The knowledge itself is considered in terms of the ethnopsychiatric theories which make the social activity itself meaningful. These theories both constitute the internal structure of the psychiatric domain and locate that domain within the larger sociocultural context of Bengal.

Chapter 1 describes the internal structure of the psychiatric domain through an examination of the psychiatric social institutions in Bengal. These institutions are considered from the perspective of the various specialists, showing their roles, norms, values, and cognitive systems as well as the physical settings in which they work. The institutions described are Western allopathic psychiatry, the traditional medical system of Ayurveda, the psychiatric activities of the ojhā [folk healers], and the temples specializing in curing psychiatric disorders.

Chapter 2 continues to explore the internal structure of the psychiatric domain but shifts attention to the clients seeking psychiatric treatment, generally for another person, the patient. The conceptual framework of the client is analyzed by identifying three paradigms of mental illness (possession, sorcery, and head malfunctioning) and by analyzing their relationship to the concept of pāgalāmi.

Chapter 3 then examines the processes by which the clients enter the psychiatric domain and initiate interaction with specialists. I view the treatment-seeking process as the development of strategies for managing the psychiatric diversity existing at the institutional and the conceptual levels. First, I examine the entry processes by which clients determine that treatment is needed. Second, I show how clients construct accounts of the search for therapy which make particular treatment-seeking choices reasonable and rational.

Chapter 4 concludes the analysis of the internal structure of the psychiatric domain by examining its pluralistic character. Relationships between the various subsystems are described in terms of competitive, particularistic, assimilationist, and inclusive relationships.

Chapter 5 introduces the second part of the study, the analysis of the psychiatric domain in the larger context of Bengali society. I focus on the patient as the embodiment of the phenomenon pāgalāmi and on the moral meanings implicit in the concept of pāgalāmi. Pāgalāmi is identified as frustrated desire, and a theory of desire in Bengali ethnopsychology is developed.

Chapter 6 then discusses pāgalāmi as entropy, as the disintegration of order due to inadequate boundary maintenance. From these conceptualizations of pāgalāmi as frustrated desire and as entropy, I derive a Bengali theory of the person. In conclusion, I contrast the concept of pāgalāmi with the Western conception of madness.

NOTES

1. This approach draws on a number of different sources. In anthropology, a focus on cultural knowledge is found in "ethnoscience," the study of "the system of knowledge and cognition typical of a given culture" (Sturtevant 1964:99; see also Spradley, 1972). In sociology, in addition to the work of phenomenologist Schutz (1970), especially relevant is that of Berger and Luckmann (1966), the ethnomethodologists (see Garfinkel, 1967; Filmer et al., 1972; R. Turner, 1974), and some of the sociolinguists (Sacks, 1972 and 1974; Labov and Fanshel, 1977).

It should also be noted that a phenomenological approach raises the fundamental question of how the researcher is to formulate knowledge. Is the introduction of analytic categories rooted in Western science acceptable or do they distort the phenomenon to be described? My own view is that analysis of emic data is often akin to the translation process -- expressing one meaning system in the language of another. Part of the meaning is inevitably lost, but that need not invalidate the value of the translation.

2. Throughout this book, Bengali words are written according to the transliteration system given in Dimock and Inden, 1969. The one exception is the symbols used for the four letters which represent "r". Two of these derive from Sanskrit and are transliterated as -r- and -ṙ-. The other two are not found in Sanskrit and are transliterated as -ṛ- and -ṛh-. Also, Bengali consonants include the implicit "a" vowel. This has been included in the transliteration but is generally not pronounced; e.g., *bhūta* is pronounced simply "bhut." Diacritic marks have not been used in spelling proper names (e.g., place names, Sanskrit texts).

A glossary of both Bengali and Sanskrit words is found in Appendix C. It should also be noted that, within long quotes translated from Bengali to English, quotation marks are used to indicate English words or phrases used by the speaker. The original Bengali is given in parentheses, and brackets are used for inserted explanatory material.

3. A similar orientation is illustrated by Blum's analysis of "not-guilty-by-reason-of-insanity" (NGI) verdicts:

> Thus, to study NGI verdicts as socially organized products, we attempt to determine...the culturally accredited implications of stating that the defendant is not-guilty-by-reason-of-insanity. Each

> rule that we locate specifies a different set of implications that the defendant is NGI:...each [rule] constitutes a different culturally accredited set of grounds for producing such a statement....You cannot legitimately call the defendant NGI without implying that you conceive of him in such and such a way....So the decision depends on the theory that the juror invokes to interpret the evidence....The proper understanding of an NGI verdict is attained only when such theorizing is described (1970:42, 43, 45).

4. It is clear that my samples are not representative of the general Bengali population. Respondents were almost exclusively Hindu, more likely to be urban and non-agricultural as well as more wealthy, more educated, and more "modern." It is also obvious to me that the social characteristics of the respondents are correlated with their conceptions of mental illness. Thus, generalization beyond the Hindu urban lower middle class from which the bulk of the data was drawn must remain tenuous. Research based on a non-Hindu or non-urban sample (e.g., Muslim agricultural peasants) might find that mental illness is more closely connected to a sociocultural system (e.g., the religious system) other than the medical one on which I have focused.

On the other hand, however, my topic is such that the relative distribution of various conceptions and behavior is of little concern. Since the goal of the research is to provide an integrated descriptive analysis of Bengali conceptions, my inability to specify the correlations between social class and seeking treatment at a medical clinic or belief in possession, while a limitation of the study, does not seem to me to affect the validity of the findings I discuss. In this regard, I am following the techniques of "theoretical sampling" as developed by Glaser and Strauss (1967:45ff).

Part I

THE INTERNAL STRUCTURE OF THE PSYCHIATRIC DOMAIN

CHAPTER 1

The Institutionalization of the Psychiatric Domain

One of the most important characteristics of the psychiatric domain is the degree to which it has been institutionalized. These institutions, recognized and differentiated by Bengalis themselves, are structural systems of such sociological abstractions as roles, norms, values, and cognitions, as well as associations of individuals and related physical facilities.

The psychiatric system in Bengal is highly pluralistic, incorporating a number of medical subsystems, each having distinct ideologies, personnel, treatment facilities, and therapeutic techniques. Since the degree of involvement of these subsystems in the psychiatric domain varies considerably, only the four most significant are described in detail. However, all of the following subsystems are included within the psychiatric domain:

1. The allopathic medical system of Western origin has become an important medical institution in Bengal and is a major resource for psychiatric treatment.

2. Homeopathic medicine, also of Western origin, is widespread and popular in India (Leslie, 1976; Bhardwaj, 1973). However, in contrast with allopathy, psychiatry has not developed as a specialization within this system. While homeopathic practitioners treat psychological disturbances in the course of a general practice, there are no homeopathic facilities in Calcutta which exclusively treat mental illness.

3. Bio-chemic medicine is a system which stresses the importance of "salts" to maintain health. It is the least institutionalized of the subsystems and the least relevant to the psychiatric domain. Bio-chemic drugs, such as kali-sulph and natrum-mur, are typically dispensed by nonprofessionals who have no formal training. They are used for minor ailments.

4. An Indian version of psychoanalysis was developed by G.S. Bose and has become quite popular throughout India. Though psychoanalysts need not be trained in allopathic medicine, it is nonetheless closely aligned with allopathic psychiatry. Therefore, I have treated psychoanalysis as a school within allopathy rather than as an independent subsystem.

5. The Ayurvedic medical system derives from ancient Sanskrit texts. Few Ayurvedic facilities and professionals presently specialize in treating mental illness, but Ayurvedic theory provides the dominant conceptual orientation to mental illness for most Bengalis.

6. Islamic or Unani medicine was brought to India around the thirteenth century. One of the most popular texts among modern Unani scholars is Avicenna's tenth-century Arabic text, itself related to the second-century Greek medical thought of Galen. Ayurveda and Unani have remained distinct subsystems, but over the years, practitioners have exchanged many ideas and therapeutic practices (Basham, 1976). Most of my respondents were Hindu and none reported consulting a hākima or Unani doctor.

7. Folk medicine, the medical activities of folk healers (ōjhā), is an important subsystem within the psychiatric domain.

8. Religious rituals and pilgrimages to temples often invoke the divine power of the gods and goddesses to cure

illness. I located two temples which specialized in the treatment of mental illness.

9. Astrologers are sought not only as advisers (e.g., regarding marriage), but also as experts in augmenting or mitigating the influence of stars and planets, which can affect health. Astrology has only minimal relevance to the psychiatric domain.

10. The philosophical-religious system of Yoga has principles which are used either to maintain mental health or to cure mental illness. Recently, several allopathic psychiatrists have taken an interest in using Yogic techniques with psychiatric patients, and one Bengali psychoanalyst has integrated Yogic meditation into his treatment procedures. However, Yoga is not a common treatment for mental illness.

Allopathic Psychiatry

> It takes about an hour to go by train from Calcutta to the small town where we met Dr. Dasgupta (a pseudonym). An allopathic psychiatrist who generally works in Calcutta, Dr. Dasgupta comes to his family home outside Calcutta two Sundays a month to run an outpatient clinic for the surrounding villages. From the train station, we took rickshaws for the 20-minute trip to Dr. Dasgupta's house. At present, no one lives there other than a few servants who keep the place in order. It is quite a large compound, with an extension off to one side which serves as the outpatient clinic. There was already a fair-sized gathering waiting for Dr. Dasgupta, and some called out greetings and even reached to touch his feet in respect as he went by.

> We were first taken into the sitting room in the main part of the house, where we were served tea. Dr. Dasgupta then ushered us to the clinic part of the house, spread a clean bed-cover on the floor for us to sit on, and ordered all those peering in at us to go away. He himself, along with a clerk who kept records, sat at a desk in another room of the clinic. Our room was very open, with several doors and windows opening to the veranda where the patients waited. In spite of Dr. Dasgupta's injunction on entering, the room soon became quite crowded. After Dr. Dasgupta finished talking with a patient and the accompanying relatives, he then directed them to talk with me. As I took a case history of the patient, there was generally little concern with the audience around us. In a couple of cases, persons in the audience added details to the history. This lack of privacy, even in the presence of the patient, embarrassed no one. Those who had finished talking with me typically joined the audience to watch interviews with others.

Allopathic psychiatry is the most institutionalized and bureaucratic of the psychiatric subsystems. Even though its intellectual roots are in Western medicine and some allopathic psychiatrists received training in England, allopathic psychiatry in Bengal still cannot be equated with psychiatry in the West. A wide variety of facilities provide allopathic treatment (Chakraborty, 1970). These include those with only inpatient services; those with only outpatient services; those with both inpatient and outpatient services; private nursing homes; and jails (see Table 2).

The two largest psychiatric hospitals for Bengal are located near Ranchi, in the neighboring state of Bihar.

TABLE 2
Allopathic Psychiatric Facilities in Bengal

Facility	Established	# beds	Outpatients/wk
Inpatient only (Ranchi)			
1. Hospital for Mental Diseases	1918	600	*
2. Ranchi Mansik Arogyashala	1952	1650	*
Jails			
1. Dum Dum Central Jail Psychiatric Unit	n.a.	880**	--
2. Lalgola Special Jail for Lunatics	n.a.	700	--
3. Vagrants' Home	n.a.	1500***	--
Inpatient and Outpatient			
1. Hospital for Mental Diseases - Gobra	1967	250	250
2. Lumbini Park Mental Hospital	1940	200	150
3. Bhowanipore Mental Observation Ward	1807	50	150
4. Calcutta Medical College/Hospital	1939	12	200
5. R.G. Kar Medical College/Hospital	1933	10	150
6. Mankundu Psychiatric Clinic	1933	200	n.a.
7. Antara	n.a.	80	n.a.
Outpatient Only			
1. National Medical College/Hospital	1964	--	100
2. G.S. Bose Clinic	1948	--	n.a.
3. N.R. Sirkar Medical College/Hospital	1962	--	n.a.
4. Ramakrishna Mission Seva Pratisthan Hospital	n.a.	--	n.a.
5. Kumar P. N. Roy Hospital	n.a.	--	n.a.
6. B.R. Singh Hospital	n.a.	--	n.a.
7. Urban Health Center, Chetla	n.a.	--	n.a.
8. City Welfare and Health	n.a.	--	30
9. Bankura Psychiatric Clinic	n.a.	--	70
Private Nursing Homes			
1. Bangiya Unmada Ashram	1935	100	--
2. Harmony Home	1967	20	--
3. Lake View Home	1965	20	--

There are at least 10 more private nursing homes in Calcutta, and two outside Calcutta.

*The outpatient clinics are rarely used by Bengalis.
**Approximately 600 are non-criminal lunatics.
***It is estimated that sixty per cent are mentally ill.

The Hospital for Mental Diseases - Kanke was originally established in the colonial period and is now run by the Central Government of India. Of its 600 beds, 260 are reserved for patients from West Bengal, at a charge of Rs. 500 to Rs. 600 per month. The grounds are spacious and attractive, and the hospital provides occupational, recreational, and behavioral therapy, as well as some psychotherapy. Nearby, the Ranchi Mansik Arogyashala, supported by the states of eastern India, has nearly 1,700 beds, almost all of which are free. Six hundred beds are reserved for West Bengal, but, since 550 of them are presently occupied by chronic patients with little hope of release, only 50 beds are available for short-term acute patients. Insufficient funds and the high number of chronic patients create a grim atmosphere in stark contrast with the peaceful quiet of the Central Government Hospital. The rehabilitation of patients is a realistic goal for the Central Government facility, while the former simply provides custodial care for the majority of its patients. The Ranchi hospitals have become so well known in Bengal that the colloquial expression, "he should be taken to Ranchi," is a way of disparaging a person's mental competence.

Within Calcutta, the major allopathic institutions are the Hospital for Mental Diseases - Gobra and the Lumbini Park Mental Hospital, private institutions which receive substantial aid from the government of West Bengal to provide free beds. Both hospitals avoid patients who might become chronic, and the average length of stay is six to eight weeks. They operate daily outpatient clinics for less severe disorders and for follow-up treatment needed by former inpatients. Lumbini was founded by the Indian Psychoanalytic Society, but no long-term psychoanalysis is currently done there. Chemotherapy and electro-convulsive therapy are the primary therapeutic techniques used, though Gobra also uses some behavior therapy.

Other facilities in Bengal specifically for the residential treatment of the mentally ill are Bhowanipore Mental Observation Ward (the oldest psychiatric institution in India), Mankundu Psychiatric Clinic in Hoogley District, and the Antara hospitals for the economically destitute, run by the Missionaries of Charity. In addition, two general hospitals in Calcutta have small inpatient wards, and there are at least 13 private psychiatric nursing homes in Calcutta. The latter are small, expensive, and run by allopathic psychiatrists who are attached to other hospitals. Outpatient services are available at Gobra and Lumbini Mental Hospitals, a number of general hospitals, and some independent outpatient clinics such as the G.S. Bose Clinic run by the Indian Psychoanalytic Society. Individual allopathic psychiatrists often have a large private practice on an outpatient basis.

Mental patients are also found in several jails. The largest of these are the Dum Dum Central Jail Psychiatric Unit (880 patients), just outside Calcutta, and the Lalgola Special Jail for Lunatics (600 to 900 patients) in Murshidabad. By virtue of the Lunacy Act of 1912, an individual can be declared a "non-criminal lunatic" and committed to the jail by order of a magistrate.[1] Originally, detention in the jail was to be temporary, until a bed became available at one of the psychiatric hospitals. However, the reluctance to admit additional potentially chronic patients presently makes transfer unlikely. Release is conditional on a magistrate's order and the family's willingness to accept responsibility for the individual. One psychiatrist estimated that several hundred patients continue to be held only because of their families' refusal to support them. A similar situation exists at the Vagrants' Home of the West Bengal Department of Social Welfare. Of the 1,500 residents, 900 are estimated to be chronically mentally ill (Chakraborty 1970:95).

The staffing at these various facilities varies, but all adopt a medical orientation. Lumbini has one government psychiatrist, five consulting psychiatrists, three resident physicians, one administrator (also a physician), one registrar, one pathologist, one physical therapist, and a nursing staff of 25. The nonprofessional staff includes aides who are responsible for the routine care of patients. In general, non-psychiatric physicians supervise the daily functioning of inpatient facilities, and psychiatrists act as consultants. Nurses and social workers are rarely trained in psychiatric treatment, and the psychologists who are occasionally part of clinic staff are restricted to administering psychometric tests. Thus, most of the staff at these allopathic facilities lack formal training in psychiatry and are familiar with the psychiatric setting only through experience.

In contrast, allopathic psychiatrists with a Diploma in Psychological Medicine (DPM) generally have two years beyond the basic medical degree. The M.D. - Psychiatry is a more advanced degree, one year beyond the DPM. In Bengal, only Calcutta University offers both the DPM and the M.D. - Psychiatry, while the Institute for Post-Graduate Medical Education and Research has a DPM course. Most Bengali allopathic psychiatrists have a DPM from Calcutta University, though a few obtained this degree from Ranchi or were trained in England. In all, 40 to 50 allopathic specialists practice in Bengal.

Typically, allopathic psychiatrists work in several settings. A particular specialist might be on the staff of a government hospital, see outpatients once a week at a smaller clinic, and have a private practice. They are hard-working and conscientious, but often defensive about local facilities which they fear would be considered inferior to those in Europe or the U.S. Those who had trained or worked in Great Britain tend to be especially apologetic, complaining about the frustrations of practicing psychiatry where facilities are ill-equipped and trained personnel inadequate. From my rough estimates, which exclude private patients, 40 to 50 psychiatrists are responsible for over 4,000 inpatients and 1,500 outpatients in any given week. It is not unusual for a psychiatrist to see as many as 20 patients in a single morning's outpatient clinic.

This specialist-client ratio is a major factor in the types of treatment used. Allopathic psychiatrists rely on drugs as the primary therapeutic intervention, regardless of their views on the causes of mental illness. Electric shock therapy is also commonly used, and desensitization behavior therapy with mild electric shocks is used at two facilities. Generally, the allopathic psychiatrists favor "supportive" psychotherapy, but little agreement exists about what this involves. Three of the 24 psychiatrists I interviewed were also psychoanalysts and two others were receiving training. At the other extreme from the psychoanalysts who might provide hour-long sessions twice a week was the psychiatrist who explained that supportive psychotherapy involved speaking with the patient once or twice a week for five or 10 minutes during routine rounds. A more typical pattern was to have 30-minute sessions once a week over a period of three to six months. Generally, psychiatrists viewed supportive therapy as giving the patient a chance to talk about current problems. While a few denigrated the efficacy of psychotherapy, most of the psychiatrists saw it as a component of an ideal treatment plan. However, in the context of the outpatient clinic or the inpatient hospital, it was unlikely that a patient would receive psychotherapy. Therefore, the few patients who did receive such therapy were almost invariably private patients who could afford to pay a substantial fee.

At Bhowanipore Mental Observation Ward, I observed more than 120 psychiatric interviews, which were typical of interviews that I observed randomly at other clinics.[2] For the new patient, the psychiatrist elicited an unstructured report of the problem through open-ended questions such as "what happened?" or "what's the problem?" This report was then followed up with direct questions regarding past episodes of mental disorder, history of mental illness in the family, and current social situation. While the psychiatrist only occasionally inquired about early childhood experiences, sleeping and eating habits were inevitably discussed. Finally, the patient would be given a prescription and asked to return, usually in two weeks. The maximum time spent with any one patient was 30 minutes, and the average time was considerably less. For return patients, the procedure was similar, though briefer, and questions concerned the time period since the last visit. Relatives nearly always accompanied the patient, and were never asked to leave so that the patient could speak with the psychiatrist alone. In fact, questions were usually directed at the relatives rather than the patient. Thus, except for the absence of a physical examination, the psychiatric outpatient interviews that I observed were identical to those one might experience in a general medical clinic in Calcutta.

Although they acknowledge differences in the actual practice of psychiatry in India and the West, Bengali allopathic psychiatrists view Western psychiatry as the model for their own. They distinguish between psychosis and neurosis, and use standard diagnostic categories (e.g., schizophrenia, endogenous depression, phobic reaction). They view disturbances as disease entities identical to those of the West. Differences, such as variation in hallucinatory content and the predominance of somatic symptoms of anxiety, are considered irrelevant to the disease process and therefore to the therapeutic intervention required. Social factors such as general public ignorance and family rejection of chronic patients may be viewed as hindering the therapeutic goal, but they are seen as peripheral issues to be remedied with greater public education. The social environment of Bengal is acknowledged as a problem at the practical level of providing service, but not as a factor requiring a fundamental reorientation of the theoretical postulates of Western psychiatry.

The range of views on the etiological factors contributing to the development of mental illness is quite wide (see Table 3). Some allopathic psychiatrists believe that mental illness is an exclusively physiological or bio-chemical process: "As a physician, I always believe that there is some biophysiological cause of mental disorder which has not yet been explored." Others profess that psychodynamic factors are the exclusive cause of mental illness. Most of the allopathic psychiatrists, however, recognize that both of these factors are etiologically important. There is a tendency to view

TABLE 3
Orientation to Etiology:
Bengali Allopathic Psychiatrists

	physiological 1	2	3	psychological 4	5	mean
Psychiatrists (N=24)	3	4	9	7	1	2.96
Psychoanalysts (N=8)	0	0	2	4	2	4.00
Total (N=29)	3	4	10	9	3	3.14

Scores were obtained by coding open-ended responses.

The three individuals who are psychiatrists with psychoanalytic certification are included in both groups.

genetic or physiological influences as providing the preconditions for mental illness with the precipitating factor located in the environment. Similarly, many agree that biochemical aspects are more significant in psychosis. Neurosis is not usually seen as the initial stage in the development of a more severe disorder, except where the physiological precondition is present.

In considering what kind of psychodynamic and environmental influences are important, some stress early psychosocial circumstances and personality development. One of the attending physicians at Lumbini Hospital told me, "Strict discipline, overprotection, puritanical attitudes: these early childhood experiences are more important than the present situation. Rome was not built in a day." Others take the opposite view and emphasize the patient's more recent circumstances, using the concept of stress. The source of stress is occasionally the family, but is more often located within the general social milieu: "We live in a competitive society and they are getting very frustrated. They always find competition and so there is anxiety and sometimes guilt. It is a social problem -- mental illness." Socioeconomic factors -- general poverty, or relative deprivation -- are often identified as a cause of distress, while frustration is a recurrent theme in the allopathic psychiatrists' statements, whether it is the result of economic conditions, job and career contingencies, or unrequited love. Most Bengali psychiatrists agree that "to relieve the poverty and frustration is most important."

Several concluding observations about allopathic psychiatry can be made. First, the allopathic facilities are concentrated in and around Calcutta, and most patients come from that area. Second, the clientele of the outpatient clinics is generally the urban lower middle class, but also includes patients from the urban lower classes and from the more affluent rural population of the neighboring districts. Third, because most outpatient clinics are either free or charge only a nominal fee, cost is not a primary consideration in the use of these facilities. Fourth, allopathic psychiatry is integrated within the general allopathic institutions, and psychiatrists must first obtain a basic medical degree. In this sense, allopathic psychiatry represents a specialization within the larger allopathic medical subsystem. Fifth, psychoanalysis has had a fairly strong influence on both the facilities available within allopathic psychiatry and the cognitive orientation of the specialists themselves. Finally, the specialists follow the model of Western psychiatry and emphasize the dual role of physiological and psychosocial processes in the development of mental disorders.

Ayurveda

> The Ayurvedic clinic run by Shri Chatterji (a pseudonym) is a 10-minute walk away from the main part of the town. Shri Chatterji was quickly informed of our arrival and we were ushered into his office. Even though his English was not very good, he insisted on speaking in English in response to my Bengali. His father had also been an Ayurvedic doctor, and in 1954 they had started this clinic specifically for the psychiatrically disordered. In the early days, his practice seems to have flourished: not only were the 30 beds full, but the veranda was converted to provide additional space. Now, however, no one came.

> His remaining three patients had been abandoned by their families many years ago. Since his son had not chosen to become a kavirāja, Shri Chatterji was planning to close the clinic as soon as he could make arrangements for the three patients. He would then move to Calcutta to live with his son.
>
> He was obviously sad as he relayed this history to me. His family had been kavirāja for generations and, while he acknowledged that his son had made the correct choice, he also indicated his sorrow at seeing the family tradition lost. When I asked him to tell me some of the Ayurvedic views on mental illness, he asked that we go to the study where he kept his books. He immediately pulled out a copy of the ancient text of *Caraka*, found the appropriate passage, and began reading it aloud in Sanskrit. Perhaps the expression on my face communicated that I understood no Sanskrit, because he stopped and told me that, to understand Ayurveda, I really must learn Sanskrit. When I said that I was familiar with *Caraka* in an English translation, he chided me that it was not the same. He then began again reading the Sanskrit. Every so often he would stop and haltingly translate the passage into English. If I stopped him to ask questions, he would hold up his hand and inform me that all I wanted to know was in *Caraka*. Eventually, he gave me some of his own interpretations and practices, but most of our visit I spent listening to him read the ancient text. As I left, he told me how glad he was that I had come because perhaps American interest in Ayurveda would help it to regain its old prestige.

Ayurveda, literally "the science of long life," derives from ancient Sanskrit literature (see Filliozat, 1964; Jolly, 1951; Kutumbiah, 1962; Sharma, 1972; and Zimmer,

1948). Just as allopathic psychiatry is not equivalent to psychiatry in the West, current Ayurvedic belief and practices are not identical to those of the ancient texts. However, to place this discussion in its sociohistorical context, I will outline the evolution of Ayurveda and its classical theory.

Ayurveda developed and flourished several centuries before Christ (Basham, 1976). The oldest text, the Caraka Samhita, was probably compiled in the first century A.D. and introduced the basic premise that health requires a balanced state of the tridoṣa [three humors: bile, phlegm, and wind]. The other major text is the Susruta Samhita (fourth century A.D.), which includes surgical techniques not discussed in Caraka. A third Ayurvedic work, Vagbhata's Astrangahdaya, dates from the seventh century A.D. There are similarities between the Ayurvedic system and the Greek medical thought of Galen (second century A.D.), indicating contact between the two, but the direction of influence is unclear (Filliozat, 1964). In any event, by the eighteenth century, "the traditional beliefs and practices of Ayurvedic physicians were radically different from the classic texts" (Leslie 1976:356).

In 1822, the School of Native Doctors was established in Calcutta, combining instruction in indigenous and Western medicine.[3] It signaled a series of debates among different British factions as to the proper approach to Ayurveda. The Anglicists favored education along European lines while the Orientalists wished to revive indigenous institutions while at the same time incorporating them within a modern scientific orientation. The Orientalists were to have a tremendous impact on the later development of Ayurveda: their interest in Indian culture became the stimulus for the Ayurvedic revival of the late 1800s and early 1900s. In 1835, while surveying medical facilities in the Nattore district of Bengal, William Adams found only one medical school, a traditional Ayurvedic _tola_ in the home of two Ayurvedic practitioners (_kavirāja_, or "king of the verses"). Ten years later, Thomas Wise published a detailed description of Ayurveda and concurred with Adams' recommendation that such indigenous institutions should receive the full support and encouragement of the colonial government. The Orientalists argued that Ayurveda had suffered a recent decline, due at least in part to the impact of Muslim and British rule and the consequent support of rival medical systems. The goal, they argued, should be to restore Ayurveda to its place of eminence in Bengali and Indian society.

Although this view of Ayurveda as experiencing a recent loss of prestige and popularity is undoubtedly distorted (Leslie, 1973), medical revivalism became associated with the general Indian renaissance of that period, and later "was also an occupational version of the nationalist ideology that evolved in middle- and upper-class urban society" (1973:229). In Bengal, the movement to revive Ayurveda was spearheaded by two famous _kavirāja_, Gangadhara Ray and Gangaprasad Sen, and their respective students (B. Gupta, 1976). In 1832, Ray organized an association of Vaidyas, the traditional caste of the _kavirāja_, and a few years later he founded a traditional _tola_ in Berhampore. His major influence was through his students and his "purist" orientation to Ayurveda. He believed that the future of Ayurveda lay in returning to the classic purity of the Sanskritic texts. On the other hand, Sen had a more "integrationist" view, wishing to combine Ayurveda with Western medicine. He himself led the burgeoning professionalization of Ayurveda by establishing fixed prices for consultations and for drugs, in direct contrast to the traditional emphasis on individualized treatment. He also began the first Bengali-language Ayurvedic periodical, Ayurveda Sanjivani.

Beginning in the mid-1800s, two main developments can be discerned in the development of Ayurveda. First was growing professionalization, pushing Ayurveda along the lines of Western medicine in terms of institutionalization. In 1878, Chandrakishore Sen began to manufacture and sell pre-prepared Ayurvedic drugs. The first Ayurvedic college in Bengal, the Calcutta Ayurvedic Institution, was founded in 1915; three more were organized within the next seven years, two of which still survive. The second trend was the continuing debate between the purists and integrationists. What is significant, however, is that both groups saw the advantage of acquiring a professional institutional structure. "The...purist pole of the dialect encouraged professionalization by justifying a reciprocal modernization of tradition to compete with the integrationists" (Leslie 1973:230). Two of the colleges represented the purist philosophy, even though such large educational facilities indicated a clear abandonment of the traditional ṭola system.

These developments in Bengal paralleled those at the national level. In 1923, the Usman Committee Report recommended an integrationist and professionalization stance, calling for the development of Ayurvedic teaching and clinical institutions. In 1948, the Chopra Report reiterated this recommendation. By 1958, there were 76 Ayurvedic colleges and the number had increased to 115 by 1972. With the national medical revivalism, Leslie argues that:

> Ayurveda...[has] evolved in an ambiguous para-professional relationship to cosmopolitan medicine....Cosmopolitan medical institutions have depended upon the professionalization of indigenous medicine to meet a substantial portion of the expanding need for professional care (1976:365-66).

Psychiatry may have been a specialization within Ayurveda in nineteenth-century Bengal. B. Gupta (1976:369) makes a brief reference to the Chittagong and Khandarpara schools of East Bengal (Bangladesh) as concentrating on the treatment of insanity. One of the Ayurvedic practitioners I talked with reported that his father and grandfather had had a flourishing practice in Chittagong. The father of another had a psychiatric clinic in Faridpur, while the 100-bed nursing home Bangiya Unmada Ashram in Calcutta had provided Ayurvedic treatment until the death of the kavirāja several years ago. Outside Bengal, the Ayurvedic Research Unit of the National Institute of Mental Health-Bangalore was established in 1963 and transferred to the Central Council for Research in Indian Medicine and Homeopathy in 1971. There I was told that the Ayurvedic treatment of mental illness was relatively common throughout South India and especially developed in Kerala.

While it is difficult to determine whether there has, in fact, been a decline in Ayurvedic psychiatry in Bengal, it is clear that present facilities are minimal. The three major general Ayurvedic clinics (Shyamadas Vaidya Shastra Pith, Astranga Ayurveda College and Hospital, and the Regional Research Institute-Ayurveda) said that they would treat mental illness, but acknowledged that few psychiatric patients actually came for treatment. I could locate only two kavirāja who specialize in treating psychiatric disorders. One was the man described earlier who had only three chronic patients. The other, a man in his sixties, had left his family's psychiatric clinic in Chittagong and now ran a general private practice with very few mental patients. In other words, I could locate no actively practicing Ayurvedic psychiatric specialist in or around Calcutta.

Classical Ayurvedic theory postulates that the world is composed of five elements: earth, water, fire, air, and ether. All food is made of these elements, their combination yielding six tastes: sweet, sour, saline, pungent, bitter, and astringent. When food is digested, it is transformed through "cooking" [i.e., heating by internal fires] into the seven bodily components (dhātu): food juice, blood, flesh, fat, bones, marrow, and semen. During this digestive process, certain waste products are also produced, including the three humors or doṣa, known in Bengali as vāyu, pitta, and kapha [wind, bile, and phlegm, respectively]. While all of the waste products are beneficial to the body in proper amounts, in excess they become "polluting agents" which disrupt health by acting on the body. Thus, health is seen as a harmonious equilibrium of the humors, and disease is due to a derangement of the humors. The specific kind of disease depends upon the particular humor which has become disrupted and the specific effect on the various dhātu.

Both Caraka and Susruta identify a distinct group of ailments as mental diseases because of their primary effect on the mind or mana (Weiss 1975:9ff).[4] The four disorders within this category are: unmāda [insanity, mania, psychosis]; bhūtonmāda [ghost madness, insanity caused by a spirit]; apasmāra [epilepsy]; and murcchā [sudden loss of consciousness, fainting]. The two primary etiological factors involved in unmāda are the consumption of prohibited, spoiled or unclean food, and attack by gods, sages, or brahmans. In addition, there are three conditions which predispose an individual to _unmāda_: terror and exhilaration of the mind, chaotic mental struggling, and limited awareness. These causes and conditions then produce certain pathological consequences for the body. "Toxic impurities pollute the heart which is the locus of intellect-judgement (_buddhi_)" and they "travel via a circulatory system...to the mind where they cause confusion" (Weiss 1976:18). The symptoms of _unmāda_ include hallucinations, clouded consciousness, disturbed vision, loss of affect, loss of memory and intellect-judgment, and violation of moral codes. Six different types of _unmāda_ with more specific etiologies and symptoms are differentiated in the texts: those caused by deranged wind, bile, or phlegm; those caused by the derangement of all three humors; those caused by sorrow and grief; and those caused by poisons. The prescribed treatment for _unmāda_ aims to restore the mind by purifying the body of the defective humors. The texts emphasize dietary restrictions and herbal medicine, but recommended treatments also include oil massage, enemas, purgatives, and fumigation by inhaling the smoke from certain burning substances. In extreme cases, "flagellation and giving shock to his mind, intellect, and body are advised" (_Caraka_ 6:9:29; quoted in Weiss 1975:18).

Both of the Bengali Ayurvedic specialists I spoke with continually emphasized that everything I wanted to know could be found in the Sanskrit texts. They professed strict adherence to the texts. While they lamented that much knowledge had been lost over the centuries, and that the present text was merely "lecture notes," both practitioners felt they were applying the ancient doctrines. At the same time, they emphasized that Ayurveda is thoroughly compatible with Western medical practice.

The *kavirāja* were quick to point out that *rauwolfia serpentina*, an Ayurvedic treatment for insanity, was the basis for the recent development of psychotropic drugs such as thorazine.

Both Ayurvedic specialists began by asserting that mental illness is the result of humoral imbalance. One *kavirāja* divided *unmāda* into two types: the violent where wind and bile are defective, and the silent where phlegm is deranged. He pointed out that humoral imbalance causes the disruption of *srota* [pathways, sometimes appearing to refer to blood vessels and other times to nerves]. Two major causes of such imbalance, he said, are the eating of incompatible foods (such as meat and milk) and worries or thoughts (*cintā*). Elaborating on the latter, he stated that "excessive thoughts are of prime importance." One example of such excessive thoughts, he told me, is the conflict between modern and traditional ideas, wherein an individual believes in ideas that he cannot implement in today's society. Other examples were frustration caused by ambition for the unattainable, and the meditational techniques of Yoga. Such excessive thoughts are also responsible for mental illness among students:

> They study too much and their nerves are very weak. Often they are from families who never had the chance for studies and now they have the opportunity. But often the students can't get good food and their nerves become weak. Weak nerves may also come from jealousy and over-ambition. Disease and some hereditary conditions can also cause weak nerves.

The other *kavirāja* did not differentiate between types of *unmāda*. In his opinion, all mental illness is the result of abnormal wind. Wind is characterized by its dryness and by its movement. It is what makes the blood circulate in the brain through minute veins. Around these veins, according to the kavirāja, are slippery membranes of phlegm which lubricate the veins and enable the blood to flow. With an excess of wind, the phlegm membranes are dried and blood circulation becomes sluggish, causing the person's normal consciousness to become impaired and pathological mental symptoms to arise. However, the ultimate cause of such symptoms is not the humors, but rather "various mental upsets (āghāta)," such as loss of all one's money, the death of a dear relative, or the separation of man and wife. In all these situations, where a disruption occurs "without reason, the nerves become shattered and then the person's resistance is reduced. The weakness of the nerves then affects the balance of the humors" because sleep, diet, and the bowels are upset. Both kavirāja, then, stress the complex interrelationship between psychological and physiological phenomenon.

In treating mental illness, both kavirāja advocate dietary restrictions and use herbal medicine to restore the humoral balance and to strengthen the nerves.[5] One uses a special nasal medicine which he blows into the patient's nose through a narrow tube. Sometimes vomiting is induced and purgatives given to purify the system. Medicated oils are often rubbed on the body, especially the head. Violent patients, one specialist said, must be exposed to the sun. He also noted that it was important to increase the patient's lucid periods: "A man is not mad 24 hours [a day]. In his lucid period, the patient must be encouraged. When he is not, he must be dealt with firmly."

In concluding this discussion of Ayurveda, the divergence between classical texts and present-day practice must be emphasized. Psychogenic factors which were ignored in Caraka and Susruta are now emphasized and integrated into the tridoṣa theory. Second, despite the resurgence and professionalization of Ayurveda in the early 1900s, facilities and personnel for the Ayurvedic treatment of mental illness are almost nonexistent. This observation is contrary to Gould's (1965) finding that "village medicine" is used for "chronic incapacitating dysfunctions" as well as Obeyesekere's (1976) more recent conclusion that Ayurvedic treatment has become a last resort for chronic psychiatric patients in Sri Lanka. Finally, it must be stressed that the lack of Ayurvedic psychiatric facilities does not imply that Ayurvedic treatment is not used in the home. On the contrary, a vulgarized version of Ayurvedic theory constitutes one of the three basic paradigms for interpreting mental illness.

Folk Psychiatry

> Before I met the *ōjhā* in the village of Dishergarh, several acquaintances warned me that he was a dangerous man who could gain control over people. When I met him, I was struck by his impressive presence. His eyes were very intense, almost hypnotic, and his speech was more a series of pronouncements than a conversation. The children were clearly frightened of him and would not venture onto the veranda where we talked. After a while, he offered to teach me some of the sacred verses he used, if I would accompany him to an abandoned Kali temple on new moon night several days later. When I asked why he was willing to communicate these verses to a woman and a foreigner, he explained that I must have been an apprentice *ōjhā* in a former life. Why else would I have come thousands and thousands of miles and seek him out in a remote Bengali village? Obviously, he said, I was drawn by my need to complete my training and it was therefore his duty

> and responsibility to teach me. On the designated night, I waited for him for several hours, but he never appeared. To my disappointment, I left India three weeks later without having learned any of the sacred verses.

The term "folk psychiatry" is used to refer to the psychiatric activities of the folk healers known in Bengal as ojhā, rojā, or guṇina. While the psychiatric relevance of the allopathic and Ayurvedic specialists is linked to conceptions of mental illness as a physiological process, folk psychiatry is included because of the belief that mental illness can be caused by possession or sorcery.

Folk psychiatry is probably the most prevalent of the psychiatric subsystems in Bengal, but also the least institutionalized.[6] Bhowmick (1973), in a survey of Midnapur District, located 462 ojhā of "high reputation." When I arranged to visit a village near Santiniketan, three ojhā agreed to talk with me while two others refused. Middle-class Bengalis assert that ojhā are only to be found in villages, but in one Calcutta slum I easily contacted two ojhā. Thus, evidence shows that folk psychiatry is prevalent and easily available.

The social characteristics of ojhā vary considerably. Bhowmick's 1973 data show that they come from a variety of caste groups and are found within the tribal and Muslim communities. The largest group (42.4 percent of the total) comes from the Mahishya caste, the most populous caste of that area. All of the ojhā in Bhowmick's sample were male, though of different ages. Most of the ojhā also engaged in some other occupation: of the six I interviewed, two were full-time practitioners, two had urban jobs, one cultivated his own land, and one was an agricultural day-laborer. Often, the ojhā does not expect any fee for his services.

Bhowmick states that the most common practice is to present some betel nuts at the time of the consultation. Later, the recovered patient may present the _ojhā_ with a piece of cloth or some money.

An interesting aspect of the folk psychiatry system is the existence of a semi-institutionalized system of training and certification. Of my sample, three had been taught by their fathers, while three had non-kin _guru_ [teachers]. Both of the professional _ojhā_ had spent two to three years with their _guru_. The majority of the _ojhā_ in Bhowmick's sample had spent over three years in training. Curiously, "there is no restriction for a higher caste member to get his training under a lower caste Guru" (Bhowmick 1973:14). The training period is initiated through a ceremony in which the student presents the _guru_ with a piece of cloth. Thereafter, the _guru_ teaches the student various _mantragupti_ [hidden or secret magical verses] and how to use magico-herbal medicines. During this period, the student is expected to adhere to certain restrictions and to worship particular deities or spirits. The disciple must also vow not to reveal the details of the training except to suitable students. Finally, training is completed with a ceremony known as _utarāna_ [passed or certified] during which the _guru_ feeds the student from his own hand.

Ōjhā engage in a wide variety of activities. Bhowmick listed 15 different specializations, and most _ojhā_ claimed proficiency in three or four areas. The treating of snake bite is the most common area of expertise. Non-medical activities include locating a lost object, identifying a thief, and generally insuring good luck and prosperity. Within the medical sphere, _ojhā_ also cure chronic diseases such as arthritis or dysentery, repair bone fractures, and induce milk supply for new mothers. Within the psychiatric domain, the ojhā have the ability to drive away ghosts (bhūta) and to counteract sorcery (tukatāka). Bhowmick's data suggest that exorcism is a common specialization among ojhā.

Among the ojhā I interviewed, five claimed to cure ghost possession. The sixth said that he did not believe in ghosts; he believed that patients said to be possessed had been affected by dūṣita hāoyā [bad or faulty wind]. The others also felt that "bad wind" is itself a factor in possession. One ojhā told me, "if a new mother or pregnant woman is struck by wind at this time [early evening], then she will be struck by apadṛṣṭi [possession]." The ojhā generally agreed that

> if a bhūta catches [i.e., possesses] someone, he will become another kind [i.e., act very differently]. When the bhūta possesses someone, the person possessed will do all sorts of trouble at home. After the bhūta leaves, he will be all right again.

Only three of the six admitted that they could perform or cure sorcery (tuka). One ojhā bragged that he could make people do whatever he wanted them to do. Another was an obvious source of anxiety in his village. Bhowmick indicated that expertise in performing tuka is relatively rare, since only 34 of the 462 ojhā claimed involvement in three sorcery-related areas: killing an enemy, making a person "mentally restless," and bringing someone under the ojhā's subjugation.

The ojhā practice a variety of therapeutic techniques, most of which fall under the category of mantraśakti, the power of magical verses. Almost any treatment procedure is accompanied by a mantra or verse believed to have extraordinary power. Medicine (oṣudha), to be consumed orally or to be rubbed on the patient, is a common form of treatment. For example, jala paṛā [literally, water reading] refers to the recitation of a mantra over water, which is then given to the patient to drink. Incense and mustard oil are also commonly given with the ubiquitous mantra. Jhāṛa phuk refers to a ritual where the ōjhā blows on the patient's body. All of these techniques can be used to cure possession, the goal being to "chase away" the offending spirit. The sacred mantra are believed to frighten the ghost into leaving the patient's body. The ōjhā may also negotiate with or badger the bhūta. Countering sorcery also requires the incantation of the powerful mantra. The ōjhā may provide the patient with an amulet (māduli or kavaca) to prevent further possession or sorcery. Worn around the neck or on the upper arm, amulets are common even among middle-class urban Bengalis. To perform sorcery, the ōjhā may prepare a potion (also called medicine, oṣudha) for the victim.[7] The ōjhā may also cast spells using the victim's hair, fingernails, or other body wastes. Bāṇamārā [literally, striking with an arrow] is another technique for performing tuka: the ōjhā uses an arrow to pierce a roughly drawn figure of an enemy.

Folk psychiatry is distinctive in a number of ways from either allopathic or Ayurvedic medicine. It has virtually no formal organizational structure and has not assumed a Western bureaucratic form the way that Ayurveda has. Also, because folk psychiatry is only one aspect of the activities of the ōjhā, it is only quasi-medical. Its link with the medical sphere is evident through the use of certain standard medical terminology: the patient (rogī) is given treatment (cikitsā) such as medicine (oṣudha) that will produce a cure (sārā). However, folk psychiatry is also firmly rooted in certain supernatural beliefs about sorcery and possession. Whereas both allopathy and Ayurveda are based upon conceptions of the individual as a psycho-physiological entity, folk psychiatry focuses on the persons's susceptibility to the influence of the occult -- ghosts and the spells of sorcerers. Outside that realm, ojhā admit their lack of expertise: "If nothing I do works, then it is a brain problem that I cannot cure."

Curing Temples

> When I visited the Kali temple at Tirole, I was very careful to dress conservatively, wearing the red-bordered white sari appropriate for a Bengali wife. My nephew accompanied me and we found that the pilgrims were very willing to talk with us. However, after four days, the priest informed my nephew without explanation that I was not to return. When I returned that afternoon to the nearby town of Arambagh where I was staying with a relative (who worked with the Public Works Department of the State of Bengal), he promised to speak with one of the leading landowners of the area who was also a distant relative of the temple priest. In the meantime, my daughters and husband arrived from Calcutta. Two days later a huge procession proceeded to the temple: myself, my husband, my daughters, my nephew, my relative and his small daughter, the landowner, and another friend. The four adult men argued heatedly with the priest for almost an hour, but he was adamant in his refusal: I was no longer welcome.
>
> In retrospect, it seems that a number of factors contributed to the priest's response. First, the teacher who had been an intermediary in establishing contact with the temple had consulted the hired priest and not the owner-priest, an

> affront to the latter's status and authority. Second, my role as a Bengali wife did not provide an adequate explanation of my presence at the temple: dutiful Bengali wives remain at home. Third, my nephew, who had grown up in a village, had nevertheless begun to wear the longer hair and jeans of the urban youth. Finally, both my nephew and I made the mistake of inquiring about financial matters. I asked pilgrims about the fees for performing rituals, and my nephew, who was also assisting my husband in his research on land tenure, asked local villagers about the temple's extensive land holdings. Since there had been recent public concern over tax evasion by temples, this inquiry into the temple's financial matters represented a threat. From the priest's point of view, a young radical and a strange American with ties to government officials were collecting potentially damaging information. No wonder I was no longer welcome.

Attributing disease to the work of deities is not uncommon in India. In Bengal, the goddess Sitalȧ is credited with causing smallpox (Nicholas and Sarkar, 1976; Bang, 1973) Other deities are believed to have the power to cure illness and restore physical health. The Kali temple at Kalighat in Calcutta and the Siva temple at Tarakeswar (see Chakrabarti, 1973) are the most popular ones for pilgrims seeking relief from disease. While mental patients may be taken to any of the temples, two Kali temples in Hoogley District are specifically for supplicants suffering from mental illness.[8]

The temple of Tirole is located in a small village three or four miles from Arambagh. On the bank of the village pond is a small Kali temple, believed to have been established in the seventeenth century because of the dream of a local Brahman. The present temple is owned by the descendants of the founder and appears relatively new and well kept. It consists of an open-sided, covered veranda, a small semi-open porch-like room, and the small inner room for the five-foot image. The goddess is called "Kapa Kali" [Mad Kali] and is jāgrata [awake], a particularly potent form of Kali. The temple is well known even in Calcutta. One of the priests estimated that 20 to 25 pilgrims come each week, either to seek treatment or to present offerings in gratitude for being cured. In the five days I was at the temple, 14 patients visited, two of whom were returning after being cured.

The Chakrapur temple is also located near Arambagh, but is only known locally. According to the present owner, the temple was founded "before the British period" when a local lord gave some land in exchange for tax-collecting services.[9] The temple for Kali was built at that time, but the treatment of mental illness was begun only 100 to 150 years ago by the owner's great-grandfather. The Chakrapur temple is substantially larger than the one at Tirole, but it is also older and now quite dilapidated. Like the Tirole temple, it sits on the bank of a pond, but it is some distance from the neighboring village. The owners of Chakrapur are low-caste Hindus (Majhi) and consequently the temple is neither as prestigious nor as wealthy as Tirole. A Brahman priest is hired to perform the rituals. The Chakrapur temple has no image of the goddess except at Kali pūjā time in October, when a special idol is set in the temple and then immersed in the pond after the ceremonies. During the rest of the year, the "life" of the goddess rests in an ordinary looking stone. Curing ceremonies at Chakrapur are held only once a month, on the night of the new moon. When I visited, a general fair was also being held and, though a good-sized crowd had congregated, only eight patients had come for treatment.

The Tirole temple has two owner-priests and a hired priest, while Chakrapur has two non-priest owners and a hired priest. No rationale for the various treatments was provided other than that they are the wish of Kali as revealed by the men who began the curing rituals. It is Kali who has the power to cure and the priests are simply her instruments. As one priest noted, "All is [according to] the Mother's desire. Why it [the illness] happens, why it becomes better -- I know none of this."

Treatment procedures at the two temples are quite similar. Both serve clients regardless of religion, and both emphasize the curing of mental illness. The supplicant, having consumed no food or drink that day, must first bathe in the adjacent pond. A pūjā or worship ritual is performed and the patient is given an iron bangle (bālā) to wear. At Tirole, the daily pūjā involves offerings of flowers and sweets, but goats are provided on new moon nights and on special occasions. At Chakrapur, goat offerings are given each new moon night; eight goats were slaughtered the time I witnessed the pūjā. After the ceremony, the patient must observe dietary and other restrictions. The cost of the bangle at Chakrapur is Rs. 11.25 plus a small fee for the priest. At Tirole, there is no fixed fee for the bangle, but several clients told me that they paid over Rs. 25, and as much as Rs. 50.

At Tirole, there are specific rules regarding the wearing of the bangle. Men must wear it on their upper right arm. Unmarried women and women whose husbands are still alive wear the bangle on their left wrist, while widows are required to wear it on the upper left arm. Menstruating women and those who are in a period of ritual mourning cannot be given the bangle. The patient is also given the blessed flower offerings and an amulet. Each day, the patient must drink the water in which these flowers have been soaked. When the flowers can no longer be used, the patient washes the amulet in water and drinks that. When the illness has been cured, the amulet must be worn around the neck or on the upper arm. A woman who is menstruating must not wear the amulet to the *ghāṭa* where dead bodies are burned or to the *ā̃tura ghaṛa* where babies are born. Hindu patients are not allowed to eat at a mourning feast (*śrāddha*) nor can they eat *boāla* fish, garlic, chicken eggs, or he-goat meat. For non-Hindus, the only dietary prohibition is beef. When cured, the patient must return for another bangle (*ārogyo bālā*) made of copper, silver, or gold. The *pūjā* ritual is again performed and any vows (*mānasika*) must be fulfilled.

At Chakrapur, the emphasis is on dietary restrictions. The day before receiving the bangle, the patient must eat vegetarian food (*nirāmiṣa*, which excludes eggs, garlic, onion, and lentils as well as meat). For 15 days after receiving the bangle, the patient must follow the same dietary regulations as widows, eating only one meal a day of vegetarian food he himself has cooked. For the first seven days, fried or baked foods are forbidden, as are leafy vegetables (*śāka*) and a particular sour drink called *ambala*. Every new moon day for a year, the patient must fast completely. Additionally, for a year's time, there are prohibitions on eating duck or chicken eggs, he-goat meat, garlic, onion, and certain fish (*śola*, *boāla*, *śiṅgi*, and *pũṭi*). Eating food cooked by persons of another caste, and eating at a ceremonial house (*karma bāṛī*), are also prohibited for a year.[10] Finally, for the first year, the patient should not be in contact with smoke from a funeral pyre, should not enter the birthing room, and should not touch women who are menstruating.

Kali is a popular goddess in Bengal, intimately connected with Tantric worship. None of the priests could provide any reason why Kali should be credited with curing mental illness. It is not a question that is relevant to their frame of reference: Kali is simply all-powerful. However, two popular myths surrounding the goddess perhaps suggest the association between Kali and mental illness.[11] In the first, Lord Siva is grieving due to the death of his wife, Soti. In his grief, he is dancing madly with her dead body, bringing destruction to all around. The other gods decide that Vishnu must bring an end to his dance by cutting up Soti's body with his discus. The pieces of Soti's body are believed to have fallen throughout India and are now the sites of particularly holy Kali temples. This myth thus pictures the Kali temples as having emerged from the cessation of madness. In the second myth, Kali herself has become mad in her fight against various demons, and is destroying innocent people. Siva, her husband, is asked to calm her down. To do so, he throws himself at her feet so that she steps on him, an incredibly shameful thing for a wife to do. The typical Kali image in Bengal portrays this scene, with Siva at Kali's feet and Kali sticking her tongue out in disgust as she is shocked to her senses by what she has done. This image of Kali is therefore a striking portrayal of madness arrested. Both myths thus link Kali to the termination of mental illness.

Role Relationships in the Psychiatric Domain

These four psychiatric subsystems -- allopathic psychiatry, Ayurvedic psychiatry, folk psychiatry, and curing temples -- are most involved in the treatment of mental illness in Bengal. Bengalis distinguish each of these subsystems and recognize their relevance to mental illness. Sociologically, each subsystem is an institution with a distinct set of roles and normative expectations. In some instances, these role expectations are the same for each subsystem, but there are also some important differences.

All of the four psychiatric institutions are organized through the interaction between persons occupying three major roles: specialist, client, and patient. The major normative expectation for each role specifies its relationship to the treatment process: the client requests treatment, the specialist provides treatment, and the patient receives treatment. Thus, the client who approaches the specialist requesting treatment is generally not the patient. Of the 120 allopathic psychiatric interviews I observed, all but two patients were accompanied by a relative who assumed the client role. In all settings I observed, most of the verbal interaction was between the specialist and the client. The individual's deep embeddedness within the kin group in Bengali society means that things often considered private in the West are considered the province of the family.

It is the client's prerogative to determine whether interaction with a specialist will take place. The client both initiates and determines whether to continue the role relationship. This expectation is extremely significant because, in the context of the pluralistic diversity of specialists, it indicates that choice of treatment is a problematic concern for the client. Once interaction has been initiated, however, the client defers to the specialist. The asymmetrical authority of the relationship dictates that the specialist will determine the nature of treatment to be provided. The client can refuse to follow recommended treatment procedures, but such a refusal is at least a partial rejection of the specialist's authority.

The authority of the specialist role derives from the practitioner's socially recognized knowledge of the psychiatric domain. However, the various subsystems view that knowledge differently. To a large degree, the authority of the allopathic psychiatrist is based on expertise and recognized effectiveness in meeting the patient's needs.[12] In contrast, the priest's knowledge derives not from any particular instrumental information or proficiency, but from a generalized attitude of devotion which enables him to mediate the relationship between the goddess and the patient. The folk healer's authority involves both devotion to a personal mentor and expertise in the use of the powerful sacred verses. The Ayurvedic specialist also seems to represent a combination of expertise and devotion. While an attitude of devotion to the ancient texts is still very important, the professionalization of Ayurveda has emphasized the Western scientific orientation and reliance on expertise.

Access to the specialist role is restricted: practitioners must be socialized. The degree to which training and social certification is institutionalized varies among the subsystems. Allopathic psychiatry has the highest degree of institutionalized socialization, while acquisition of the specialist role in folk medicine rests on a more informal and variable process of socialization.

The priesthood is hereditary, as is ownership of the temples, but instruction is required for assuming the duties of a priest. Within Ayurveda, at one time only members of one caste group were kavirāja, but the development of a more institutionalized form of socialization has diminished the hereditary aspect of the role.

In general, then, the degree of institutionalization varies from one subsystem to another. Allopathic psychiatry has a high degree of formal structure with numerous interlocking facilities and personnel, as well as formal regulations regarding the acquisition of the specialist role. It is linked to the general institutional system of allopathic medicine, and hence to the political structure, through financial and legal regulations relating to allopathic psychiatric activities. On the other hand, the curing temples are institutionally linked to the traditional religious system. As specialists, the priests of the curing temples are regulated by Hindu doctrine and practice. Ayurveda has become bureaucratized to some extent in this century, but it still has a less complex institutional structure than allopathy. Folk psychiatry represents the other extreme -- a reliance on a more informal structural arrangement.

NOTES

1. The Lunacy Act also provides for the commitment of "Under-Trial Prisoners" and "Convicted Prisoners" to the psychiatric unit of the jail for an indeterminate length of time. The former are persons against whom a criminal charge has been brought and who are awaiting trail. The latter have already been convicted of crimes. At Dum Dum Jail, there are about 100 persons in each of these two categories.

2. My role at the clinics posed a certain ethical dilemma. Bhowanipore is both an educational and research institution where observation of psychiatric interviews was not uncommon. Nonetheless, while the psychiatrists were fully informed of my research, they never explained my presence to clients, who consequently had little idea of the role. When I began interviewing, the social worker who brought the patients to me was expected to explain that I was a visiting researcher and to ask if they objected to an interview with me. In fact, she typically just told clients that they were now to meet with me. I found that my own attempts at explanation were not successful at countering the clients' previous assumption that I must be one of the medical personnel. Naturally, all medical questions were referred to the social worker. While this was not an ideal solution, the clients' lack of an accurate understanding of my role was not, I feel, detrimental to their welfare.

3. My discussion of the later development of Ayurveda relies heavily on the work of Charles Leslie (1967, 1973, 1974, and 1976). For an account of Ayurveda in nineteenth- and twentieth-century Bengal, see B. Gupta, 1976.

4. I am indebted to Mitchell Weiss for providing me with copies of his unpublished manuscripts, from which I am borrowing extensively.

5. After returning from the field, I located an article by a Calcutta kavirāja entitled, "My Experiments with Cuckoo's Meat in the Treatment of Mental Diseases." He claims to have treated over 2,000 mental patients and he argues that derangement of pitta [bile] is the primary causative factor. He recommends a soup of cuckoo-meat because "it is a killer of Pitta, increaser of semen, intelligence, intellect, and a restorer of lost energy, strength, and vitality" (Chatterjee 1972:81).

6. For accounts of folk medicine in other parts of India, see Carstairs, 1955; Gould, 1957 and 1965; Hasan, 1967; Khare, 1963; Marriott, 1955; Opler, 1958 and 1963; Beals, 1976; Berreman, 1964; Epstein, 1974; Harper, 1957 and 1963; and D. Kakar, 1972.

7. Bhowmick cites the following procedure to induce insanity:

> The magician will catch or collect a Hilsa fish, unhurt. It will be buried underground on a Saturday (New moon). It will be there for one month. Then it will be unearthed. Due to decomposition, it will be infested with worms. All these worms will be dried up in the sun. These will then be pounded and diluted with water, which will be kept in a corner of the house. A fragrant flower will be dipped into it at night, and then the smell of the flower, it is said, will make a man completely mad (1973:17).

8. Temples for curing madness are probably found throughout India. Somasundaram (1973) describes several Vishnu and Siva temples in Tamil Nadu to which mental patients are brought.

9. Ralph Nicholas suggested in conversation that this most likely refers to the Nawab Nazim of Bengal, who gave out temple land in that area in the seventeenth century.

10. "Ceremonial house" or karma bārī refers to the home of a family where one of the various rites of passage (saṃskāra) is being performed: sādha [during pregnancy], annaprāśana [first rice eating], paita [sacred thread ceremony], biye [marriage], and śrāddha [funeral].

11. My thanks to Aditi Nath Sarkar for bringing these myths to my attention. It must be remembered, however, that not all Kali temples stress the curing of mental illness.

12. In actual practice, the authority of the allopathic specialist is also derived from general social status. Brahmans are overrepresented among the allopathic psychiatrists. This fusing of authority is certainly important, but it does not contradict my assertion that the authority of the role itself derives from knowledge.

CHAPTER 2

Cognitive Conceptions of Pagalami

The institutional structure of the psychiatric domain in Bengal constitutes the world of the specialist. This world includes other social actors such as colleagues and clients, particular physical settings such as clinics and temples, and customary therapeutic behavior such as writing prescriptions or reciting _mantra_. It also includes a set of cognitive conceptions which specialists use in the course of their psychiatric activities, concepts like schizophrenia, _tridoṣa_ and _tukatāka_. While clients participate with specialists in these institutional structures, they do not necessarily share the specialists' cognitive conceptions. This chapter explores the world of the client and especially the client's cognitive orientation.[1]

Three Paradigms

While I began my research by focusing on the Bengali word _pāgalāmi_ [madness or mental illness], I soon learned that three phenomena were subsumed under this term: _bhūta bhara_ [ghost possession], _tukatāka_ [black magic or sorcery], and _māthāra golamāla_ [malfunctioning of the head]. These constitute the three paradigms used by Bengalis to interpret madness.

Several terms are used to signify possession, the most common of which are _bhūta bhara_, _bhūte pāoyā_ [the getting or receiving of a ghost], and _apadṛṣṭi_ [literally, inauspicious glance]. Possession need not refer to ghosts, but can also involve gods and goddesses. In the latter case, possession typically occurs during religious festivals, bestows a sacred or occult power (śakti) on the individual, and is not related to pāgalāmi.

Bhūta are dead persons who linger in this world because they died "before their time." Suicide and accidents are common examples wherein death might result in the individual becoming a bhūta. Jaggi (1973a:183) also mentions persons who are attached to wealth, children, and other material objects; those who die with unfulfilled sexual cravings; persons with an intense hatred of someone; and those who have been murdered. In one story told to me, a woman who died in childbirth became a bhūta because of her attachment to her newborn child. Also, those whose funeral rites have not been completed are likely to become bhūta. In all cases, the person who died has not found release from the material world because of a continued emotional attachment to it.

Belief in bhūta is widespread. Children from more affluent families often have books with stories of ghosts and the havoc they cause for the living. Everyone is fond of relating stories which describe how they were almost caught by a bhūta. Older children often tease younger ones by sneaking up on them at night and talking in the characteristically nasal voice that all recognize as belonging to a ghost. It is usual for people going out at night to take some precaution to protect themselves from the roving bhūta, the most common being uttering a mantra or wearing iron. Similarly, because ghosts are so often found there, people are likely to take similar precautions when going near cremation grounds and nima trees.

Generally, vulnerability to possession seems to depend upon being in the right place at the right time. No particular group of people was identified as being more susceptible to possession than another. When I suggested that a sinful person might be a likely victim, the ōjhā disagreed, saying that such a person has sufficient power to fight off a bhūta. However, Jaggi (1973a) does note that persons in a state of ritual impurity are highly vulnerable to possession.

As illustrated in the sample interview given in Appendix B, the major symptom associated with possession is the transformation of the individual's personality. Since the bhūta takes over the body of the possessed person, possession is suspected when an individual suddenly begins to act in an uncharacteristic manner. An ōjhā described possessed persons as being "of another kind." For example, a young girl was thought to be possessed when she threw a bucket of water at her father-in-law, a serious offense for a new bride that was, her father reported, totally out of character for his well-brought-up daughter. Because of the increased power (śakti) of the bhūta, the patient's strength (also śakti) is said to increase tremendously. Hostility and aggression are thought to be especially indicative of possession.

A dramatic example of this assumption of a new personality was a young girl who became possessed by her husband's sister, who had died several years before. She began addressing her husband as dādā, older brother. When asked how he knew the girl was possessed, the ōjhā replied, "the patient described the pretātmā's [self of the dead person] life history, her love affairs, and everything.

She told how, at 12 years of age, she [the husband's sister] had been bitten by a fox."

Another common symptom of possession is rigidity. Bhūta are believed to catch their victims by the back and are said to be "riding" them. My assistant witnessed the possession of an ōjhā's wife:

> In front of our eyes, an incredible incident occurred. As the ōjhā was relating stories, his wife was sitting on the bed very normally. Suddenly, she began to shake -- hand and foot. Her eyes stared without blinking, her mouth shut tightly, and her body was rigid. Stopping his story, the ōjhā got up and went next to her. The ōjhā lit incense and held it in front of her eyes. On her eyes and mouth, he sprinkled blessed [mantrapūta] water. He covered her eyes and face with her sari. He bent the rigid arm. The ōjhā offered homage to god. He asked his wife, "Will you say something?" There was no answer. Because of the incense, her eyes teared a great deal. Gradually, five minutes later, her eyes closed. When the ōjhā was holding the incense, he told us to say "There is peace." He told us, "There is nothing to be afraid of. This happens often. Brahma has possessed her."

Sorcery is the second phenomenon included under pāgalāmi. Sorcery is referred to as tuka or tukatāka, but more often alluded to with a phrase such as "someone fed him a potion (oṣudha, medicine)." Like possession, sorcery is a category which extends beyond pāgalāmi. It can include disease of any kind as well as accidents and various misfortunes, such as failure in school examinations or lack of career advancement. Also, like possession, belief in sorcery is common even among educated Bengalis.

Not all disease, however, is attributed to sorcery. Because the human being is subject to physiological disturbances such as humoral imbalance, sorcery is used as a residual category. Two factors provoke suspicions of sorcery. When there is some abnormality in the disease which does not fit the expected pattern, then sorcery is used as an explanatory category. But since sorcery-caused illnesses mimic natural ones, anomalies are hard to detect. Therefore, a better indication of tuka is that the illness does not respond to the appropriate treatment. An ex post facto logic is used to conclude that "since the patient has not been cured by the doctor's medicine, then the problem is not illness, but sorcery."

In the psychiatric domain, sorcery can mimic māthāra golamāla. But it can also cause personality change. Such change is akin to that of possession, but the significant factor is that the person acts against his or her own interests. The new bride who becomes hostile toward her husband is a possible victim of tuka because she "obviously" respects and honors him. Her hostility must therefore be the result of sorcery designed to turn the husband's feelings against her. Similarly, when a man becomes enamored of a woman other than his wife, it is thought that another is performing black magic to ruin him. Such violations of Bengali "common sense" can be explained only in terms of sorcery (see Geertz, 1975).

The second factor which generates accusations of foul play is the existence of someone with animosity toward the victim. Feelings of jealousy or envy are especially associated with sorcery. A business rival, a jealous co-worker, a rejected lover -- all are possible agents of tuka. An infertile woman is often an object of anxiety because of her possible jealousy of other women with children. In general, it is improper to praise a child because it might indicate the speaker's envy of the child's good qualities, and imply malice toward the child. While sorcery is generally regarded as deliberate, the sterile woman's longing for a child is believed to be so strong that it can unintentionally cause harm.

Accusations of sorcery are especially common when a young bride acts strangely. By custom, the bride lives with her in-laws, and almost anyone in that household might be suspected of ill will toward her. The mother-in-law may envy the attention her son now gives his wife; brothers-in-law may be jealous of the respect and devotion the bride accords her husband; the husband may still long for a previous lover. Wives of the husband's brothers are particularly suspect: the competition and hostility among sisters-in-law can generate envy of the new bride's good qualities and jealousy of perceived preferential treatment in the family. Other researchers (Opler, 1958; Harper, 1963; Freed and Freed, 1964; Beals, 1976) have noted that possession is common among new brides; I believe, however, that in-laws use possession to explain psychological disturbances because they can thereby avoid speculating about sorcery among themselves. The girl's natal family, which might suspect sorcery, is usually from a different village and may not become involved if the episode passes. Furthermore, accusations of sorcery are likely to disrupt relations between the two families and thereby jeopardize the in-laws' goodwill, perhaps even forcing the termination of the marriage relationship. In my experience, accusations of sorcery are likely only if the in-laws have returned the bride to her own family. At this point, the wife's family can point to sorcery, to lessen the shame associated with the return of a bride.

A woman who brought her married daughter to an allopathic clinic voiced her suspicions of sorcery:

> Her head became frog-bad.[2] Her intelligence is a little weak. From her own inclination, she does not work. If told to work, she has no sense of responsibility. That's why she was thrown out of her in-laws' house. Before her marriage, there was not that much [irresponsibility]. We thought that if she gets married, she will be cured, but it seems to have increased. It seems that some _tukatāka_ was done. I took her to see _ōjhā_. They said that the boy [her husband] is being influenced by a girl [a lover]. They [the in-laws] fed her something. They cut some of her hair [for performing _tuka_]....The _ōjhā_ say that some body dirt [_gāyera mayalā_] was taken and something fed to her, in order to drive her away. The _ōjhā_ could not do anything.

The third phenomenon, _māthāra golamāla_, is also referred to as _māthā-khārāpa_ [bad head], _māthā-garama_ [hot head], or even _unmāda_ [insanity]. These terms all have a variety of implications depending on their situated use, but each can refer to the concept or cognitive category that I will label _māthāra golamāla_. _Māthāra golamāla_ entails a conception of the body as the site of various physiological processes, processes which can become disturbed to produce disease. _Māthāra golamāla_ is one such disease, the malfunctioning of processes located within the head.

Bengalis generally recognize the Ayurvedic theory of the three humors and their role in disease. They also accept the Ayurvedic doctrine that dietary regulations are intended to produce a balanced state of the body (Beech, 1976). The ideal meal is expected to incorporate the six tastes: sweet, sour, saline, pungent, bitter, and astringent. For example, a meal might include bitter melon, a salty portion of fried vegetable or fish, a pungent curry, a sour mango preparation, a sweet rice pudding, and astringent betel nuts. Consuming meals involving all six tastes enables a person to maintain the proper balance of the three humors.

However, while the three-humor system is known and used, Bengalis more commonly refer to the single dichotomy of "hot" (garama) and "cold" (ṭhāṇḍā), which refer to the humors pitta [bile] and kapha [phlegm]. Meat, eggs, onions, garlic, and one variety of lentils are the primary respresentatives of hot foods, and dairy products and most vegetables are cold. Similarly, all diseases are placed into one of these two categories: a stomachache, for example, is hot, while pneumonia is cold. Furthermore, food restrictions are inevitably a part of the treatment for any illness. Cold diseases are treated by feeding the patient hot foods, and vice versa. For example, a person with head congestion would be given plenty of meat and eggs but prohibited any cold food such as milk, which would stimulate the production of the phlegm. Conversely, a patient with stomach problems would be treated by encouraging dairy products and avoiding hot, bile-producing foods such as meat.

This hot-cold distinction can also be applied to the temperament of individuals. A person who is ṭhāṇḍā [cold] is calm, peaceful, not easily upset or angered, and generally easy to get along with. In contrast, a garama mejāja [hot temperament] individual is active, quick to anger, and anxious, and has a strong sex drive. Thus, various emotions are also labeled hot or cold: anger and sexuality are hot, while tranquility is cold. For a person to be ṭhāṇḍā is viewed as a valued characteristic, while to be garama is not appreciated. Just as food is used to affect one's physical state, it can also be used to influence one's emotional temperament. For example, vegetarian food (nirāmiṣa, which proscribes any hot food including onions and garlic) is required of widows, in order to reduce their sexual feelings, and of those who are to be participants in various religious ceremonies, in order to enhance their ritual purity.

As indicated by the colloquial term māthā-garama [hot head], mental illness is a hot disease. As such, it is attributed to excess bile, which generates excess heat. This belief seems to be the origin of the "burning sensation" complaint noted by Chakraborty (1971). She found that, while only one percent of the general medical patients exhibited such a symptom, 10.1 percent of the psychotic patients, 14 percent of the neurotics, and 35 percent of those diagnosed as having anxiety neurosis, complained of burning sensations. She interprets the symptom as the patient's way of indicating distress:

> The complaints of sensations of heat signify attempts on the part of the patients to make a diagnosis, on the basis of their knowledge of mental and physical mechanisms. Patients are trying to say through this complaint that a harmful imbalance has taken place in them and inner processes may be going out of control (1971:6).

Finally, the most common etiological factor attributable to māthāra golamāla is "shock." Among nonspecialists, the typical answer to the direct question, "how does pāgalāmi occur?" is "if one receives a shock, one will become mad." The English word "shock" may be used, even by those with little knowledge of English, or the Bengali terms śoka or manera āghāta may be used. The latter can be translated as "upsets of the mind," while the former refers to grief, especially that associated with the death of a loved one. Even when the English "shock" is used, death of a loved one is frequently cited as an example of "shock." Other examples are failure in examinations, business or career failures, rejection by a lover, and inability to have children. Grief, like sexuality and anger, generates heat and disrupts the functionings of the body's humors. In this way, the physical and psychological processes are seen as integrated. Emotions, physiology, and dietary customs are all mutually interdependent. Bengalis feel not only that "you are what you eat," but also that "you are what you feel."

Interviews with the relatives of patients at allopathic clinics provide frequent descriptions of māthāra golamāla:

> Four months earlier he had a fever. After that, his head was on fire [jvālā kare] and he spoke a lot of nonsense [bak-bak]. Then, he would stay sitting silently. He said that his head became hot. Then his head was rinsed. And oil rubbed.

> It began in 1952; her head became bad. Just after we came from East Bengal, my two brothers had smallpox. Three or four days later, they died. Mother [the patient] also had pox....And since then, this has happened.

> It began due to studies. She was studying philosophy honors when the first attack happened. In her higher secondary examination in logic, she did not get "letter marks" [an excellent grade]. This was the first setback.

> We think that after four miscarriages this happened. Because with no children to see, her "affection" became so much that from that her reason (bojhā) has gone. That's the cause.

Table 4 summarizes the distinctive characteristics of the three phenomena: bhara [possession], tuka [sorcery], and māthāra golamāla [head malfunctioning]. As demonstrated by the table, each of the paradigms is quite distinctive in terms of treatment and etiology, but overlaps and converges with regard to symptomatology and prognosis.

Pāgalāmi

The Bengali word pāgalāmi can best be translated as "madness" or "craziness," with the adjective pāgala signifying "mad" or "crazy." Like the English term "crazy," pāgalāmi can be used in a number of different contexts. It can be applied to some non-serious disturbances of no psychiatric relevance, as in sentences such as "literature is his pāgalāmi" or "if this heat continues, I'll become pāgala." Second, pāgalāmi can refer to a description of observable behavioral phenomena or the symptoms associated with psychological disturbance. Third, the term may be used to identity a specific process taking place within an individual which results in such symptoms. I shall refer to these last two as "phenotypic pāgalāmi" and "genotypic pāgalāmi."[3]

The contrast between phenotypic and genotypic pāgalāmi is an ontological one. Phenotypic pāgalāmi indicates the level of sense data and of appearances; genotypic pāgalāmi refers to that of ontological existence and reality. This distinction between phenotypic and genotypic pāgalāmi should not be unfamiliar to Westerners. It is the difference between saying that a person is behaving madly and saying that a person is mad. It is the difference

TABLE 4
Three Paradigms

Paradigm	Etiology	Symptoms	Treatment	Prognosis
māthāra golamāla	"shock"; excess bile	burning sensations; hallucinations; anger;	medical: medicine and diet	variable; often chronic; relapse
tuka	envy of victim; spell, potion	mimics disease; personality change	counter spell: consult _ōjhā_	variable; permanent cure possible
bhara	chance circumstances	rigidity; aggression; personality change	exorcise _bhūta_: consult _ōjhā_	variable; permanent cure possible

between describing behavior and characterizing an individual. For example, the person who has taken a hallucinogen may be acting crazy (phenotypic pāgalāmi), but most Westerners would not say that such a person was really insane (genotypic pāgalāmi).

Similarly, among Bengalis, phenotypic pāgalāmi refers to those traits and symptoms that can actually be observed. For instance, hallucinations, inexplicable hostility, and excessive grief or withdrawal are all traits that Bengalis would identity as phenotypic pāgalāmi. A person exhibiting these symptoms would be seen as pāgala. All three of the phenomena (possession, sorcery, and head malfunctioning) may result in symptoms that Bengalis would label pāgalāmi; each, then, is seen as resulting in phenotypic pāgalāmi.

On the other hand, genotypic pāgalāmi refers to a particular underlying psychophysiological process. A person experiencing such a process would be said to be genotypically pāgala. Such genotypic pāgalāmi only refers to head malfunctioning. When discussing a person who is phenotypically pāgala due to possession or sorcery, Bengalis are apt to indicate that the person is not really pāgala, implying that it is not a case of genotypic pāgalāmi. In this sense, both possession and sorcery represent a kind of pseudo-pāgalāmi, wherein the person only appears to be pāgala. According to Bengali common sense, there are three reasons why a person might act pāgala, but only one reason a person would really be pāgala.

It should be clear that it would be an oversimplification to state that there are three causes of pāgalāmi. From the Bengali point of view, there are three ontologically real phenomena: bhara [possession], tuka [sorcery], and asukha [disease]. Each of these can result in phenotypic pāgalāmi, but they can all produce other outcomes as well. Possession can result in divine inspiration, sorcery can cause accident and misfortune, and disease can produce other physical symptoms. Only māthāra golamāla, the disease of head malfunctioning, is the cause of genotypic pāgalāmi. These relationships are diagrammed in Figure 1.

This analysis demonstrates the crucial importance for researchers to attend to the ontological assumptions behind the use of various concepts and not to project their own conceptual categories onto the terms used by others. To say that possession and sorcery are indigenous concepts of mental illness is to confuse the two ontological levels. Only māthāra golamāla as a type of disease is the equivalent of the Western concept of mental illness, at least as conceptualized within the medical model.

An example of a failure to understand this distinction between the two ontological levels is Clements' (1932) popular classification of disease causation. He argues that all cultural groups subscribe to one or more of five basic explanations for disease: soul-loss, breach of taboo, disease sorcery, object intrusion, and spirit intrusion. My analysis suggests that this kind of presentation of ethnographic data is based on the researcher's own preconceived notion of the world. The researcher may be approaching the data with the assumption that instances of illness are readily recognizable. Thus, when he examines various causes of what he *knows* to be illness, he assumes that the indigenous population also *knows* that it is disease, and thus that any distinctions made are an attempt to differentiate types or causes of disease. In other words, the researcher believes that

FIGURE 1

The Cognitive Structure of the Psychiatric Domain

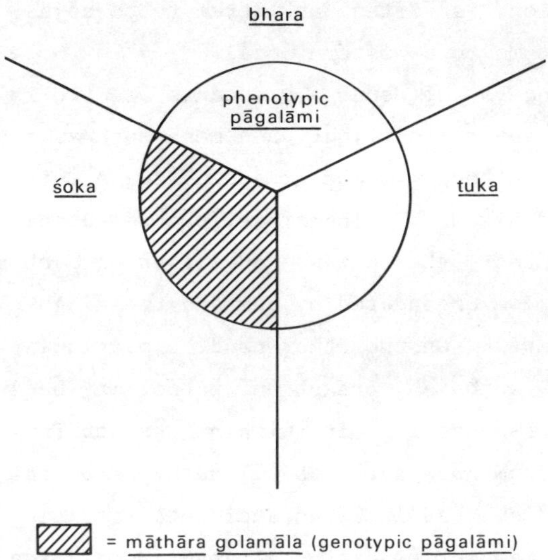

statements such as "he is possessed by a spirit" mean that "he is sick because he is possessed by a spirit." However, spirit possession may not be a cause of illness, but an alternate and contrasting phenomenon, just as bhara and māthāra golamāla are to Bengalis. Use of Clements' classification is often an attempt to adjust indigenous thought systems to a Western model.

The dangers of such a procedure are two-fold. On the one hand, several distinct phenomena such as soul-loss and breach of taboo may be reduced to a single Western phenomenon, disease. Therefore, the researcher may not be able to detect the unique qualities of each phenomenon; e.g., the awe engendered by one and the disgust associated with another. On the other hand, a particular indigenous phenomenon, such as breach of taboo, may be artificially restricted by keeping it within the confines of a given Western phenomenon such as illness. From the indigenous point of view, bad luck and accidents resulting from taboo violations may not be differentiated from "disease" that is similarly caused.

Just as ethnographers should avoid ethnocentrically imposing their own values, they must also be conscious of the problems of imposing their own cognitive system. The systematic categorization of the experiential world into "things" such as disease can be just an ethnocentric as one's value system. Thus, it is misleading to talk of indigenous "explanations" of disease if a cultural group has no conception of "disease." The concept of "disease" implies the abnormality of the organism as a biological entity, and such a perspective on human beings may be lacking. For example, Manning and Fabrega point out that the Maya of Mexico believe that "the self and the body are only diffusely distinguished in social transactions and are considered continuous. As such, both are affected by illness" (1973:261). Similarly, V. Turner has noted that "the Ndembu 'doctor' sees his task less as curing an individual patient than as remedying the ills of a corporate group" (1964:262). Thus, in these instances, to focus on explanations of disease is to gloss over significant differences in the very conception of human beings and the afflictions to which they are vulnerable.

NOTES

1. A sample interview, along with a discussion of the analytical process, is presented in Appendix B: Interviewing Clients.

2. Most Bengalis I asked had never heard of this phrase (beṅ khārāpa). One servant said that it meant that her head was bad because a frog was inside it, hopping around.

3. These terms are borrowed from the field of genetics. Genotype refers to an individual's actual gene structure and phenotype refers to the physical appearance of the individual. I am using the terms to differentiate two similar levels of "reality," that of structure and that of appearances.

CHAPTER 3

Seeking Psychiatric Treatment

The psychiatric domain in Bengal incorporates a high degree of pluralism -- pluralism both at the structural level of the psychiatric institutions and at the conceptual level of the three paradigms of pāgalāmi. This pluralism constitutes the background for the role relationship between specialist and client. Since the specialist-client relationship becomes established through the initiative of the client, the pluralism of the psychiatric domain forms the context within which clients make specific treatment decisions and engage in specific treatment-seeking behavior. How do clients come to act within the psychiatric domain and thus develop decision-making strategies which reflect such psychiatric diversity? This process of establishing the specialist-client relationship has two components: entry into the psychiatric domain and treatment-seeking. The former refers to the client's realization that the patient's situation requires psychiatric intervention. The latter refers to processes for determining which particular specialist will be consulted.

Entry into the Psychiatric Domain

The most frequent way in which a client enters the psychiatric domain is through an evaluation that the patient is phenotypically pāgala [crazy]. Because this judgment usually occurs prior to treatment-seeking behavior, the processes which affect that judgment occurred prior to my contact with clients. Thus, I shall only briefly identify three factors involved in that judgment: the characteristics of the event being evaluated; the characteristics of the actors making the judgment; and the situation within which such judgments take place.

As part of my research, I administered the Star Questionnaire (see Appendix A), a set of six descriptive paragraphs describing persons whom Western psychiatrists usually view as mentally ill. Using this instrument, it is possible to identify the characteristics which lead non-specialists to make judgments about psychological abnormality. For example, the juvenile delinquent was rarely seen as pāgala, while the unreasonable aggressiveness of the paranoid schizophrenic often prompted judgments that he was pāgala.

However, it is also clear that such personality characteristics are evaluated within two different frames of reference. In reply to the question as to whether a particular person's behavior is "abnormal" (asvābhāvika), some respondents would just shrug their shoulders and reply "some people are like that." When I presented these case histories to a group of students for discussion, the dual referent of "normal" was made explicit. "Really, there is no right answer. We could either try and see whether the person is abnormal compared with others or compared with his own nature. A person could be abnormal in one sense and not in another." This finding is consistent with Kakar's (1978) observation that psychological deviance is tolerated because of respect for each individual's unique "person nature" (svadharma, also personal code of conduct). Thus, divergence from "one's own nature" is considered more serious. For example, withdrawn behavior would be of greater concern in a previously extroverted adolescent.

Second, various characteristics of the respondents affected their judgments. Bengali psychiatrists view the young woman described in the Star Questionnaire as continually checking to see that she has locked her door as compulsive, but housewives view her as merely absent-minded. The different educational backgrounds of psychiatrists and housewives create differences in the available categories they can use, and thus result in different responses. In response to another of the Star descriptions, men are less likely than women to view a withdrawn woman as psychologically abnormal. Presumably, the cultural norm which dictates that young women behave circumspectly around men reinforces the male belief that such "shy" behavior is quite normal for women. Additionally, the interests of the various actors affect their evaluation. Because pāgalāmi can be hereditary and thus can hinder the family's ability to arrange satisfactory marriages, close consanguine relatives are probably less likely to perceive the patient as pāgala. In one instance, a medical student who had made a "love match" brought his fiancée to an allopathic clinic for treatment, stating that her illness would not affect their marriage arrangements because he was quite sure that she had only had an adverse reaction to an antibiotic. Generally, however, new brides may be more quickly viewed as psychiatrically disordered because their in-laws' home is a social context where no such interests are served in denying pāgalāmi.

Third, it is obvious that, in contrast to the artificial questionnaire judgments, evaluations of actual events and persons are socially situated. A key component of that social context is the group of actors, generally kin members, who constitute what Janzen (1978) calls the therapy management group. The final outcome involves negotiation among them, and the final decision is influenced by who is participating in the debate, their relative power relations, and the context within which the debate takes place. Again citing the case of the new bride, consanguine relatives may oppose the in-laws' attempt to assign a label of pāgalāmi, but the discussion will vary substantially depending on whether the in-laws want to return the bride or merely to obtain treatment for her. In addition to Janzen's discussion of this process in the use of African medical treatment, labeling theory has long focused on this negotiation process (see, for example, Rubington and Weinberg, 1978). While it was not a focus of my research, its significance must be acknowledged.

The social consequences of judging someone as phenotypically pāgala are clear and explicit: kin members are obliged to assume the role of client in order to provide treatment for the patients. When asked what should be done if someone is mentally ill, Bengalis responded either that treatment (cikitsā) is necessary or that the individual should be taken to a doctor. The societal response to pāgalāmi is treatment or intervention by a specialist, rather than ostracism, punishment, or some other response to deviant behavior. For a person to acknowledge that a close kin member is pāgala dictates that treatment decisions must be made. Conversely, clients can adequately explain treatment-seeking behavior simply by noting that the patient is asustha [sick] and pāgala [crazy]. It is this normative expectation and obligation to seek treatment that links the client and the specialist, establishing this relationship as the crucial one within the psychiatric domain.

In addition to the family's judgment that a patient is psychologically disturbed, another common route for entering the psychiatric domain is through referral. Typically, clients are referred to allopathic specialists by general allopathic practitioners. The charts from an allopathic clinic reveal that one criterion used by general practitioners for making a psychiatric referral is the presence of physical complaints without any identifiable physiological cause. This procedure may also explain the frequent observation by psychiatrists and researchers (Chakraborty, 1971; Chakraborty and Mallick, 1966; N. Gupta, 1956; and Rastogi, et al., 1976) that Indian patients express anxiety through somatic symptoms. The prevalence of such patients may not reflect unique psychological dynamics but rather the referral process.[1]

From the clients' perspective, this referral procedure may force a redefinition of the situation. Clients seeking treatment from a general allopathic practitioner may not perceive the patient as pāgala. In this case, clients enter the psychiatric domain only when and if they come to accept the specialist's view that the problem is a psychiatric one. Because specialists are given the authority to determine the diagnosis and the required treatment, most clients probably accept this redefinition without hesitation. But it is also possible that ignorance regarding the significance of the referral leaves the client unaware that a redefinition has taken place. Furthermore, the client may at times reject the referral and its implied redefinition of the situation. In one example, a young married woman refused to return to the psychiatrist because she was convinced that all her problems were a consequence of her inability to have children. She continued to visit the gynecologist who had referred her to the psychiatrist, and felt that she only required treatment for her infertility. In this instance, the client avoided entering the psychiatric domain and a psychiatric definition of the situation.[2]

Accounting for Psychiatric Treatment Seeking

When I interviewed clients in various psychiatric institutional settings, I began by asking, "Why did you come here?" I chose this particular question because it avoided medical terminology and provided clients with maximum flexibility to respond according to their own system of relevances. I expected that clients would describe the patient's problems as a justification for seeking psychiatric treatment in general. To my surprise, clients often responded by explaining why they chose that particular clinic or doctor or temple. The clients answered by saying that their brother-in-law recommended the temple, that their neighbor works in the hospital, or that they live nearby. In answering my question in terms of why the patient was brought to a particular specialist, clients were reacting to the institutional pluralism of the psychiatric domain. The treatment-seeking process involves an evaluation of various treatment alternatives so that a decision can be made to adopt a particular behavioral strategy. A major issue, therefore, is how one client comes to consult an _ōjhā_ while another seeks allopathic treatment.

Analytically, the responses to my initial interview question are examples of the performative use of language noted earlier, wherein speech is a means for engaging in social action and accomplishing an interactive task (Austin, 1962; Labov and Fanshel, 1977). The answers given are "accounts" (Scott and Lyman, 1968), verbal activity which provides a justification or legitimation of a particular behavior, which in this case is the clients' treatment seeking behavior.[3] Therefore, to ask clients why they came for treatment is to request an account that will explain, justify, and legitimate their behavior. As an account, the speaker's answer is not so much a portrayal of the actual reasons for a particular behavior as it is a social event designed to make the behavior meaningful to speaker and listener.[4]

From this perspective, clients' responses to the question "Why did you come here?" must be viewed as reasons which are culturally acceptable to explain seeking psychiatric treatment. As a whole, these reasons constitute a "cultural stock of knowledge" (Schutz, 1970) which describes the circumstances for which it is culturally acceptable to obtain psychiatric treatment. This cultural stock of knowledge is then available to Bengalis to perform the task of constructing an account as an answer to the question. Thus, to describe the treatment-seeking process, I am describing this cultural stock of knowledge and the cognitive structure of the psychiatric domain which enables clients to structure, verbalize, and thus account for their behavior.

The three paradigms of p̄agal̄ami described in the previous chapter are an initial presentation of the cultural knowledge available. Table 5 presents a slightly altered version of the earlier table: non-medical

TABLE 5
The Structure of the Psychiatric Cognitive System

Prior event	Genotype	Phenotype	Social action	Outcome
1. "shock"	mathāra golamāla	pāgalāmi: physiological changes; burning sensations	medical: medicine & diet	restoration of humoral balance; variable
2. envy of victim; spell	tuka	pāgalāmi: personality change; violating self-interest	consult ōjhā: counter spell	neutralization of sorcery; variable
3. attack by bhūta; chance circumstance	bhara	pāgalāmi: assume bhūta's personality	consult ōjhā: exorcise bhūta	expulsion of bhūta; variable

columns = five paradigmatic series; rows = three syntagmatic chains terminology has been substituted and the three paradigms are listed as genotypes. This presentation is more than a convenient summary; it also represents the structural arrangement of cultural psychiatric knowledge. Because they provide principles which can be used to construct accounts, the structural relations are crucial to understanding how ethnopsychiatric knowledge is used in actual social praxis.

The structure of the psychiatric knowledge system can be analyzed through the use of the concepts "paradigmatic series" and "syntagmatic chain." Paradigmatic series are constructed by grouping together items which "are associated in our minds as somehow similar in function or 'meaning'" (Leach 1970:46). In Table 5, the vertical columns represent the five paradigmatic series: prior event, genotype, phenotype, social action, and outcome. Thus, for instance, the paradigmatic series of genotypes is formed by the paradigms of tuka, bhara, and māthāra golamāla. In like manner, the other four paradigmatic series shown in the table are constructed through a recognition of similarity.

In contrast, the syntagmatic chains are constructed on the basis of contiguity so that they are juxtaposed to one another sequentially. The basic syntagmatic chain is composed of a set of paradigmatic series and the "syntax" that connects them:

prior event	(causes)
genotype	(which becomes manifested as)
phenotype	(stimulating the normative expectation to engage in)
social action	(thereby resulting in)
outcome	

Once this structural arrangement of Bengali psychiatric knowledge is understood, the problem of choosing a particular treatment alternative can now be rephrased.

What are the principles by which Bengalis justify the choice of a particular item from within the paradigmatic series of "social action"? It is my view that Bengalis can construct socially legitimated accounts of psychiatric treatment-seeking behavior by invoking four structural features of the ethnopsychiatric cognitive system.

A particular syntagmatic chain is formed by selecting one option from each of the paradigmatic series. The most critical structural feature of the ethnopsychiatric cognitive system, however, is selective restriction, i.e., certain choices from one paradigmatic series will entail the exclusion of some options in another paradigmatic series.[5] In fact, the restrictions on selections are such that only three syntagmatic chains are meaningful (represented by the rows in Table 5):

> 1. Māthāra golamāla [head disorder] syntagmatic chain: Shock (causes) māthāra golamāla (which becomes manifested as) physiological changes such as "burning sensations" (stimulating the normative expectation to engage in) medical and dietary treatment (thereby resulting in) restoration of humoral equilibrium.
>
> 2. Tuka [sorcery] syntagmatic chain: Magical practices (cause) tuka (which becomes manifested as) personality changes such as acting against one's self-interest (stimulating the normative expectation to engage in) further magical procedures by the ōjhā (thereby resulting in) neutralization of the spell.
>
> 3. Bhara [possession] syntagmatic chain: The attack of a bhūta (causes) bhara (which becomes manifested as) transformation into the bhūta's personality (stimulating the normative expectation to engage in) exorcism (thereby resulting in) expulsion of the bhūta.

Thus, the selective restrictions are such that the choice of any one item indicates a complete syntagmatic chain. For instance, "behavior against one's self-interest" implies the entire bhūta syntagmatic chain. Thus, a particular treatment choice can be justified simply by identifying the appropriate syntagmatic chain. That is, the principle of selective restrictions enables Bengalis to construct accounts for treatment-seeking behavior by citing any one of the other items in a specific syntagmatic chain.

Examples of clients using this strategy to produce accounts of their treatment behavior are common in my interview data. A husband who brought his wife for treatment told me,

> "One child died. My parents accused her. Since then, she has stayed sitting in her room....Perhaps that's why the disease happened."

Here, the husband is explaining his treatment-seeking behavior by referring to prior events -- the death of a child and accusations by in-laws -- which are viewed as "shock" and thus possible causes of the disease māthāra golamāla. In another instance, a mother did not suggest any possible causal factors, but simply indicated the genotype māthāra golamāla as a justification for obtaining treatment:

> Her head has some disturbance (golamāla). That's why I brought her here.

An additional example of an account which relies on this principle of selective restriction is the client who describes the phenotypic symptoms the patient has. Thus, a wife told me about her husband:

> Before, he worked hard. Now he only sits quietly and does no work. He is afraid all the time. His head reels. Like a mad person, he sits quietly. That's why I brought him here.

Finally, a client can account for treatment behavior by asserting that the present difficulty is a recurrence of a previous illness which had a positive outcome from similar treatment:

> It began 8 to 9 months before. ECT [electric shock therapy] was given. After that, she became better. After that, the illness again happened.

While all of the above examples use the māthāra golamāla syntagmatic chain, the principle of selective restriction similarly applies to the other two chains. For example, if I had asked the father in the sample interview (see Appendix B) why he had taken his son to see an ōjhā, he could have alluded to the bhūta syntagmatic chain by referring to a prior event known to be causally linked to possession: "A few days before, he had gone fishing and came home late." Or a client could invoke the tuka syntagmatic chain, for example, by describing the patient's phenotypic appearance and noting that the patient is acting against his/her own best interests. In every case, clients are tacitly acknowledging the structure of the psychiatric cognitive system and using it as a resource for constructing an explanation or account of their behavior.

Conversely, others in the interaction and we as observers can only understand the client by reference to the implicit syntagmatic chains which link causal event, phenotype, genotype, social action, and outcome into an ordered sequence. Because this cognitive system is not explicit and, for the most part, cannot be made explicit by

Bengali actors, it is an example of what Sperber (1974) refers to as tacit knowledge. It forms the taken-for-granted common understandings which make such statements and the behavior thereby accounted for meaningful. The reason for my inability to understand the statement about fishing in the sample interview given in Appendix B was that the bhūta syntagmatic chain was not part of my cultural stock of knowledge. It is only by reference to this tacit knowledge that Bengalis can establish what Garfinkel (1967) might call the rational-adequacy-for-all-practical-purposes of their statements and their behavior.

This first structural principle, constructing accounts by invoking one of the three syntagmatic chains, is complemented by a second: that of excluding two of the syntagmatic chains. A particular treatment-seeking behavior can be accounted for by establishing the inappropriateness of the other two syntagmatic chains. Since there are only three genotypic paradigms which can result in pāgalāmi, excluding two of them is equivalent to asserting the third. For example, a client might explain coming to an allopathic clinic by simply saying that the patient is neither possessed nor bewitched:

> [After telling of strange behavior] There is total awareness. It is not possession. All day he is fine. But from evening to morning, he is out of control.

Because it is difficult to assert conclusively that the other paradigms are inaccurate, use of this principle of exclusion is not very frequent. However, clients would often justify treatment choices on the basis that other treatments had failed. The failure of a particular treatment negates the relevant syntagmatic chain as being applicable to that case. A mother uses this technique in describing her daughter's case history:

> We thought that someone had bewitched her. We saw an ōjhā. He gave many amulets, but nothing happened. The astrologer said that her Mars and Saturn are very bad and that the wind [vāyu] was faulty. He gave an amulet. From that, nothing happened.

A third structural principle which characterizes the psychiatric knowledge system is that of cognitive indeterminacy. By indeterminacy, I am referring to the fact that the various paradigms, the cells of the table, can be expanded. For instance, there are many discrete events which would all be considered instances of "shock" and which together would constitute the paradigm "shock." That is, we could expand each of the paradigms to incorporate an infinite number of unique observable events; or conversely, there can never be a finite set of events which together constitute the entire set "instances of shock." This principle can be applied to the items within the event, phenotype, and outcome paradigmatic series.

The cognitive indeterminacy just cited in the concept "shock" is an example within the event paradigmatic series. Not only is there no determinate list of events which will have a particular result, but no event will invariably produce certain results. The probabilistic and contingent nature of causal relations is acknowledged. Going fishing at night will cause possession -- if the individual has not taken proper precautions and if bhūta have been attracted. Similarly, while bhūta are more active at night, disturbing a sleeping bhūta in the daytime is especially dangerous. This recognition of causal indeterminacy means that it is never possible to be absolutely sure that a specific event has a specific result.

Cognitive indeterminacy is also incorporated within the phenotypic paradigmatic series. While there can be distinctive symptomology associated with each of the genotypes, there is significant overlap. Anger and aggressiveness can be a sign of too much bile, a sign of the bhūta's appropriation of the victim's body, or a sign of the tuka's potency. It is this phenotypic fusion which enable all of the phenotypes to be characterized as pāgalāmi and which results in the inclusion of all three within the Bengali psychiatric domain.

Finally, indeterminacy is recognized within therapeutic treatment because outcomes are likely to vary from situation to situation. Human ability to affect the world through their actions is acknowledged as limited and contingent. For example, exorcism rituals will be effective in expelling the bhūta -- if they are done properly and if the ōjhā has sufficient strength to overpower the ghost. Similarly, medical treatment will be effective -- if the proper medicine is given and if the disorder is not so serious that it resists treatment. The failure of one particular therapeutic practice, such as a particular ritual by a particular ōjhā, does not mean that a different ritual or a different ōjhā might not be successful. Even though the hypothesis that a particular event is an instance within one of the syntagmatic chains is "tested" through examining the treatment outcome, the principle of cognitive indeterminacy means that treatment failure does not necessarily disconfirm the hypothesis. Only successful treatment can confirm the hypothesis; e.g., since exorcism cured the patient, she must have been possessed.

The indeterminacy of the cognitive system means that it is impossible either to locate or to exclude a particular syntagmatic chain in a definitive manner. Therefore, treatment-seeking behavior is hesitant, tentative, and irresolute. Conversely, an argument can always be presented to counter claims that a given psychiatric event either is or is not an instance of one of the syntagmatic chains. A father's claim that his son became possessed when he went fishing at night can be countered by saying that fishing at night might cause possession, but maybe it didn't this time; or by saying that the son's fear of his father appears to be a symptom of possession but maybe it is really a symptom of sorcery. In other words, in any specific instance, arguments can be presented for each of the three syntagmatic chains.

As a structural principle that can be invoked for constructing accounts of treatment-seeking behavior, cognitive indeterminacy is substantively different from the two earlier principles. Whereas the principles of selective restriction and exclusion can account for a particular treatment strategy, the principle of cognitive indeterminacy accounts for strategies which combine several treatment behaviors. The client's own uncertainty can prompt using several treatments at the same time. Another of the social consequences of this indeterminacy is that it permits disagreement and thus creates an arena for negotiation among those in the therapy management group which Janzen (1978) discusses. One solution to such disagreement is to use several alternate treatment strategies. Generally, in the face of such ambiguity where it is virtually impossible to establish a conclusive definition of the situation, it makes sense to try anything and everything available. Thus, accounts based on the indeterminacy of the cognitive system legitimate a multiplicity of treatment-seeking behaviors in a single psychiatric episode. As one client reported,

> There have been many treatments....[gives details] After that, I brought her here. We will do everything.

One additional implication of the principle of cognitive indeterminacy is especially striking: it undermines the use of the other two princples. That is, recognition of the fundamental indeterminacy of the system invalidates the logic which underlies the principles of selective restriction and exclusion. These principles rely on the assumption that a particular psychiatric event can be located within or excluded from the various syntagmatic chains. The principle of cognitive indeterminacy declares that assumption to be false. But significantly, this contradiction is irrelevant to social action in a fundamental way. As Garfinkel (1967) stresses, the client only seeks rational-adequacy-for-all-practical-purposes. That is, the accounts must be "rational" and "logical" only insofar as they must be accepted as adequate accounts by others. As Schutz points out, the actor

> does not search for the truth and does not quest for certainty. All he wants is information on likelihood and insight into the chances or risks which the situation at hand entails for the outcome of his actions (1970:76).

Finally, a fourth structural principle used for producing adequate accounts of psychiatric behavior is the situatedness of the psychiatric domain. Bengalis do not view the psychiatric domain as an isolated and inviolate area of cultural space. Rather, it is a part of the total social system within which the client is enmeshed, and therefore its boundaries are continually infringed upon by other considerations. The pragmatics of cost and availability are one such factor. It is quite legitimate to account for going to a clinic because it is nearby, or to account for terminating treatment because it is too expensive. Particularly given the indeterminacy of the cognitive system, it only makes sense to try the most accessible and cheapest treatments first or to stop ineffectual treatments which are expensive and difficult to obtain. In the following excerpt, a father decides not to pursue a successful treatment because it is less accessible:

> The ōjhā gave some medicine, but he is far away. That's why it is inconvenient to go. Tomorrow is the day to take him. After taking the ōjhā's medicine, he got somewhat better.

Similarly, treatment-seeking behavior can be justified by the need to maintain relationships with significant others. As a way to demonstrate honor and respect for those with superior status, it is important to heed their advice regarding treatment. It is extremely common for clients to account for their treatment decisions by acknowledging the person whose advice they were following: "Hearing of the clinic from my father, I came." Often, these social considerations are designed to affirm relationships with kin members, but any person with superior status should be so respected. A married woman explained the reason why she brought her mother to the allopathic clinic:

> My sister took mother to a sādhu [holy man] of a Kali temple. The sādhu spoke of this place and of ECT. That's why I came here.

A third area which penetrates the psychiatric domain is the religious, though in a different manner. Whereas the pragmatic considerations of cost and availability and the social considerations of sustaining proper relationships intrude into the psychiatric domain, the religious consideration of devotion to the gods can be more accurately said to encompass the psychiatric domain (see Wadley, 1975). In this context, it is irrelevant to discover the appropriate syntagmatic chain because an appeal to the gods can accomplish the desired outcome in all circumstances. Thus, a request for divine assistance as an element within the paradigmatic series of social action negates the usual selective restrictions: it is always an appropriate social action. In a sense, there is an additional syntagmatic chain, one which derives from the religious domain but circumscribes the other three: all human desires and aspirations can be achieved by devotion to the gods. As the old priest at Tirole temple aptly stated, "All is the will of Mother Kali." Invoking the inclusiveness of the religious domain to justify treatment behavior, one woman explained,

> [My husband] made me very afraid....Then in a dream the goddess Mangolacandi told me, "Gouri, you go to P.G. [the clinic]. It will be good."

To summarize, clients can construct socially adequate accounts for their treatment-seeking behavior by referring to four structural features of the cognitive system. First, that system is structured by selective restraints which permit only three syntagmatic chains. This principle of selective restriction is the most frequent basis for producing an account. Second, the exclusion of two of the chains is equivalent to asserting the third. By means of this principle of exclusion, accounts for a particular action can be made by establishing the inappropriateness of the other two alternatives. Third, the cognitive system incorporates a very high degree of indeterminacy such that a particular psychiatric event can be set within any of the three syntagmatic chains. This indeterminacy becomes the basis by which accounts of plural strategies become meaningful. Fourth, the system is recognized as situated within the larger social context. The principle of situatedness is used to construct accounts where non-psychiatric factors (cost, availability, social relationships, and divine devotion) impinge on the treatment-seeking process.

Conclusion: Accounts and Behavior

Within the client-specialist relationship, the client assumes the responsibility for initiating the relationship and therefore for seeking treatment. This chapter has explored the processes by which such treatment-seeking takes place, and has argued that these processes can only be understood with reference to the structure of the cognitive system used to account for treatment-seeking behavior.

The psychiatric cognitive system is one where choices and decisions are always problematic and tentative, but always accountable. The essential accountability of decisions derives from the structural organization and accounting principles just elaborated. The cognitive system provides the means by which a client can construct an account of a particular treatment-seeking behavior. It makes treatment-seeking strategies reasonable, rational, and accountable. Thus, the cognitive system provides a theory-constructed world within which clients' behavior can be seen as meaningful both to themselves and to others. Treatment-seeking behavior in Bengal is highly theoretic and cognitive, based upon a highly complex and developed system of cultural knowledge.

On the other hand, however, the cognitive system permits a tremendous variety of responses. The indeterminacy of the system itself means that decisions about treatment strategies are problematic. They are tentative, uncertain, and open to debate. Therefore, pluralistic strategies (either simultaneous or sequential) derive not from naivete or conceptual confusion, but from the indeterminacy of the system itself. Plastic and malleable as it is, the cognitive system of the psychiatric domain provides actors with a diverse set of categories to invoke on various occasions.

Finally, it is important to explicitly clarify the relationship between these accounts or explanations for behavior and the behavior itself. Clearly, neither the accounts nor the cognitive system on which they are based can be said to determine the actor's behavior. Psychiatric knowledge does not cause certain behavioral responses. Rather, the cognitive system provides an important context within which psychiatric treatment-seeking takes place. Cognitive evaluations regarding events, genotypes, and phenotypes establish normative expectations for certain social action or treatment-seeking behavior. Bengalis know what to do because they evaluate what various things (events, entities, appearances) are. A cognitive definition of the situation is crucial in structuring particular treatment-seeking strategies.

This analysis will not enable prediction of what treatment behavior a particular person will adopt in a given case, but it will provide the terms of the debate which will surround any such decision. Therefore, the cognitive system can be seen as the available raw material out of which clients must construct their own behavior, including accounts of that behavior. Insofar as actors desire to see themselves and to be seen by others as "rational" (i.e., as behaving meaningfully), the cognitive system does mark the constraints within which meaningful, "rational" behavior must be located. If we accept Garfinkel's dictum that "the activities whereby members produce and manage settings of organized everyday affairs are identical with members' procedures for making those settings 'account-able'" (1967:1), then the accounts and the cognitive system on which they are based provide a set of socially reasonable actions.

The relationship between knowledge and behavior is therefore not unlike that between language and speech. Language consists of the set of all possible sentences generated by a particular set of syntactic rules (see Lyons, 1970). Likewise, the structural principles of the cognitive system generate a set of meaningful social actions. If it is to be meaningful, actual verbal behavior or speech is confined by the rules of language; so too for psychiatric behavior. But one can always speak or act in a way that is not meaningful. Just as language explains but does not cause or predict speech, so does the psychiatric cognitive system explain but neither cause nor predict treatment-seeking behavior.

NOTES

1. This issue is an interesting one. Based on the responses to the case histories of the Star Questionnaire, my suspicion is that most Bengalis would not view general psychological anxiety as a matter of medical concern. Thus, persons experiencing such anxiety are unlikely to come to the notice of medical personnel until such time as somatic complaints arise. However, it is still possible -- even likely -- that Bengalis do tend to express anxiety somatically. My sense is that emotional expressions of non-specific psychological distress and anxiety are difficult for Bengalis, perhaps because such expressions are not taken seriously. From a psychodynamic perspective, it could be argued that these emotions are repressed to such an extent that they eventually find somatic expression.

2. It is also important to note, however, that a client may consult a general practitioner even though the problem is already recognized as a psychiatric one. Again, because of the authority granted the medical practitioner, relying on him/her to make a referral to a specialist is both practical and logical medical behavior. Clients often view the whole medical institution as one involving esoteric knowledge unavailable to them. And, perhaps most importantly, it is believed that relationships with high-status persons such as psychiatric specialists are best established through intermediaries who will act on one's behalf to obtain the assistance needed. The social hierarchy seems to dictate that specialists be approached through general practitioners. That the prestige of the referring doctor is considered important is evident by the common practice of presenting a note from the referring doctor which contains no medical information but which serves to "introduce" the client. In any event, the point to be noted is that recognition of the psychiatric nature of the concern and thus entry into the psychiatric domain, may have occurred prior to the referral process.

3. Scott and Lyman (1968) use the term "account" in a more restrictive sense where the actor's behavior has not been in accord with expectations. They use the term "explanations" as the more general category, equivalent to my use of "accounts." Other discussions relevant to the concept of accounts can be found in Mills's (1940) article on vocabularies of motive and in Evans-Pritchard's (1937) article on magic and sorcery. The latter was the stimulus for a collection of essays on the general theme of the

allocation of responsibility within a social system (Gluckman, 1972). My concept of "account" can also be related to Schutz's (1970:126ff) conception of motives. He makes the distinction between "in order to" motives which refer to the actor's subjective intentions and "because" motives which involve the actor becoming an observer of his own past actions. In this sense, "because" motives are equivalent to my use of "accounts." Since "because" motives derive from theories actors have about themselves and about the world, they are an excellent source of data about those theories.

4. One of the important characteristics of accounts is that they must be "adequate." That is, they must be able to accomplish the task of providing a socially acceptable justification of the speaker's behavior. Three distinct aspects of adequacy can be identified: self-adequacy, other-adequacy, and identity-adequacy. An account is self-adequate to the extent that it is acceptable to the speaker as "reasonable" and in accord with the speaker's own commonsense notions of why people do things. In the social context, an account must also be other-adequate or acceptable and reasonable to the other in the interaction. If the account is not other-adequate, the speaker is likely to be challenged and asked to give another or additional account (e.g., "I'm sorry, but that just doesn't make sense"). Ivan Karp has also pointed out in conversation that accounts often must be adequate with reference to some significant other outside the interactional sequence. Finally, accounts must also generally be identity-adequate; that is, they should be identity- sustaining so that they reinforce the particular kind of person that the actor wishes to communicate to the other.

The significance of this concept of the adequacy of accounts is the implication for analyzing conversational data. To answer a question demanding an account, the speaker must not only evaluate motivational material (why one "really" behaved that way) but also, if not primarily, the adequacy of the account. Thus, responses to the question "why did you come here?" must be treated as accounts which may or may not be representations of actual motivational events. Additionally, it should be noted that the request for an account can be put off or refused. Such responses, however, open up the actor to a restatement of the request or to a further request for an account of the put-off or refusal. Furthermore, such put-offs and refusals tend to become challenges which have the potential for signaling conflict. See Labov and Fanshel, 1977.

5. The clearest example of a syntagmatic chain is in the domain of language. The basic syntagmatic chain (i.e., sentence) of subject-verb-object can be "the dog saw the cat," "the cat saw the dog," "the boy hit the ball," etc. An example of the principle of selective restriction is the verb "saw." Since it excludes inanimate subjects, the sentence "the ball saw the boy" is not meaningful. Another example of this kind of analysis would be the food domain. A particular meal (syntagmatic chain) involves a selection for each course (paradigmatic series) on the menu: for example, tomato juice, roast beef, potatoes, peas, and apple pie. Again, the principle of selective restriction invalidates some options; in a Jewish kosher meal, the roast beef selection excludes milk desserts.

CHAPTER 4

Psychiatric Pluralism

Recent work in medical anthropology has identified pluralism as a key structural feature of many health care systems.[1] Indeed, Leslie has argued that "all medical systems can be conceived as pluralistic structures" (1980: 191). An analysis of psychiatric pluralism in Bengal will make possible an integrated view of the internal structure already described, and permit a critical examination of the concept of medical pluralism and medical structures in general.

The focus on the interaction between client and practitioner helps to clarify the three varieties of pluralism that exist within the psychiatric domain. First, the psychiatric practitioner is located within a system of institutional pluralism. Each of the four major psychiatric institutions has a distinctive theoretical perspective, treatment facilities, personnel, and therapeutic techniques. Second, the client is enmeshed within a system of cultural cognitive pluralism with three alternate explanatory models available. Finally, a third variety of pluralism results because the practitioners and clients view the very structure of the psychiatric system differently. This structural pluralism results because of the divergence between the clients' perspective and that of the practitioners.

Institutional Pluralism

The psychiatric domain includes four major psychiatric institutions: allopathy, Ayurveda, folk medicine, and curing temples. Each of these is acknowledged as relevant to the treatment of <u>pāgalāmi</u> and each is recognized as a distinct subsystem. An interesting aspect of the institutional component of the psychiatric domain is how these psychiatric subsystems relate to each other. To describe these relationships, I shall make use of Young's (1976) suggestion that three ideal typical relationships can exist within a pluralistic medical system: competition, particularism, and assimilation. To these, I will add a fourth ideal type -- inclusion.

Within an organizational structure characterized by competition, each of the components is perceived as a rival subsystem. That is, each postulates a different view of psychiatric reality which contradicts the others. The various subsystems are then fully autonomous and mutually exclusive, each competing for ideological truth as well as for clients. Adherence to one automatically involves the negation or disqualification of the claims of the others. Within the second ideal typical mode of relationship, particularism, relatively autonomous subsystems are each perceived as relevant only to a particular sub-domain (e.g., symptom, disease, or category of people). In other words, competition and rivalry are avoided by a narrow specialization which locates the focus of each subsystem. Third, a relationship of assimilation would be one where the various subsystems have lost their autonomy such that each has incorporated the others. In the ideal typical assimilation relationship, it would in fact be misleading to speak of a pluralistic system with differing component subsystems. Rather, the result would be a single undifferentiated system, even though various aspects have been derived from differing medical traditions or sources. Finally, an inclusive relationship would establish the hierarchical dominance of one system over another. Thus, one subsystem has a subordinate relationship to the other as in a paramedical role. The Bengali institutional structure involves all four of these ideal typical relationships.

Competitive relations are evident in the attitudes of many of the specialists toward each other. Allopathic psychiatrists are likely to view the other subsystems as conflicting with and antagonistic to their own. Suggestions that Ayurvedic practitioners might have an important role to play in the modern health care system were met with consternation and even indignation. Allopathic psychiatrists question the theoretical frameworks of the other subsystems and view allopathy as the only legitimate psychiatric system. They argue that early psychiatric intervention by "modern, scientific" personnel is crucial to mental health and that, therefore, the most important task is to educate the public to accept and make use of allopathic psychiatry. In some instances, other specialists also had a competitive attitude towards other subsystems. Both of the Ayurvedic specialists specifically told me that patients who had had prior electro-convulsive shock treatments probably could not be cured. One Ayurvedic <u>kavirāja</u> told me, "We do not like places like Ranchi [i.e., government mental hospitals]." Similarly, at one of the curing temples, patients were specifically prohibited from obtaining any other treatment.

However, it would be an oversimplification to say that the only relationship between specialists is a competitive one. One _ōjhā_ indicated that he would refer patients with "brain problems" to a medical specialist. Ayurvedic practitioners often stressed the theoretical compatibility of Ayurveda and allopathy: they believe that allopathy is merely a more ancient version of the scientific mode. Thermometers and stethoscopes are quite commonly used, even by village _kavirāja_ (Marriott, 1955; Gould, 1965), and Ayurvedic colleges often possess Western medical laboratories (Leslie, 1973). Western psychiatric terminology is often used, and some Ayurvedic personnel also obtain an allopathic degree. _Kavirāja_ often view the use of the Ayurvedic drug _rauwolfia_ as the basis for many modern anti-psychotic drugs as an indication that the two systems are complementary.

In their turn, some allopathic psychiatrists had an ambivalent attitude toward the other systems, especially Ayurveda and the temples. Even though the theoretical system of Ayurveda was rejected, there was still considerable interest in Ayurveda and Ayurvedic drugs. Referring to Ayurvedic techniques, the newspaper _Ananda Bazar Patrika_ quoted a leading psychiatrist as saying "the ancient Indian style of shock treatment was the forerunner of modern shock therapy." Similarly, while allopathic psychiatrists may decry corruption in the temples, they are unlikely to reject outright the fundamental religious premises on which religious curing rests. Religious activities such as prayer and meditation are sometimes advocated as forms of psychotherapy; one Calcutta psychoanalyst, for example, uses Yogic exercises with his clients. Religious principles are often seen as congruent with basic psychodynamic mechanisms: "Indian patients suffering from 'depressive illness' can benefit if the principles enunciated in the Gita are developed into a type of psychotherapy. Bhagavad Gita is a masterpiece of psychotherapy" (Ananda Bhara Patrika).

Thus, while competition is clearly evident, it does not preclude some appreciation of the other systems. From the point of view of the allopathic specialists, allopathy is the preeminent psychiatric system. Some Ayurvedic and religious principles might be worthy of incorporation, but the dominance of allopathy is an unquestioned goal. The Ayurvedic practitioners have a similar, but inverted view. Ayurveda could form the basis for a comprehensive psychiatry, assimilating the benefits of modern allopathy. However, since they are very aware that their position in the psychiatric system is a precarious one, the Ayurvedic practitioners realize that the practical task is to strive for respectability rather than dominance. They want to be honored colleagues of the more prestigious allopathic psychiatrists.

Folk healers seem to acknowledge that they have a particularistic role to play in the psychiatric domain. Sorcery and possession are their areas of specialization. A specific healer as well as folk healers in general are usually recognized as having an explicitly and narrowly defined range of competence. In contrast to this "social ecological niche" carved out by folk psychiatry, the temple priests view themselves as representatives of the religious "sacred canopy" which encompasses all of human activity. If other medical treatment is tolerated or even encouraged, it is within the context of religion's inclusive relationship to the other systems.

When we analyze these relationships among the psychiatric subsystems from the point of view of the practitioners themselves, the institutional structure is a reflection of the practitioners' attitudes towards each other. Competition tends to characterize allopathic psychiatry's relationship with the other psychiatric subsystems, although there is some willingness to assimilate Ayurvedic contributions and to respect the temple's inclusive claim. Ayurveda, in response to its lower status in the psychiatric domain, has generally attempted to assimilate conceptions and procedures from Western medicine. Folk psychiatry is basically a particularistic subsystem stressing expertise in certain narrow areas. Finally, while there is some competition, the priests of the curing temples claim an inclusive relationship. These relationships are summarized in Table 6.

Cognitive Pluralism

In addition to the institutional pluralism of the specialist, the psychiatric domain encompasses the world of the client and the client's conceptual structure. The second variety of pluralism is thus cognitive pluralism and the structural patterns that clients establish through their treatment-seeking behavior (see Table 7). Treatment-seeking strategies involve the decision to consult one practitioner rather than another and therefore structure the psychiatric institutions by channelling the flow of clients into each subsystem.

In the case of sorcery and possession, the normative expectation for treatment is consultation with a folk healer. That is, the clients' perceptions of folk psychiatry is in accord with the folk healer's own view:

TABLE 6
Structural Interrelationships:
Specialists' Views

	Allopathic View of	Ayurvedic View of	Folk View of	Temples' View of
Allopathy	-	c, a	p	c, i
Ayurveda	c, a	--	p	c, i
Folk	c	c	-	c, i
Temples	c, a, i	c, i	i	-

TABLE 7
Structural Interrelationships:
Clients' Views

	Ayurveda's Relationship With	Folk Relationship With	Temples' Relationship With
Allopathy	a	p	i
Ayurveda		p	i
Folk			i

***************************** KEY ****************************

a = assimilation
i = inclusion
c = competition
p = particularism

folk psychiatry has a particularistic relationship to the rest of the psychiatric domain. Similarly, clients, like the priests, see religion as a superordinate subsystem which encompasses the others. The legitimacy of taking patients to a temple is based upon the inclusive relationship that religion has with respect to the other subsystems.

The relationship between allopathy and Ayurveda is more complex. Clients typically use the Ayurvedically derived concept of "head disturbance" to understand and interpret mental illness. The descriptions clients give of patients' symptoms, the prevalence of the "burning sensations" complaint among psychiatric patients, and the use of Ayurvedically derived home remedies, such as pouring oil or water on the head, indicate the continuing influence of Ayurvedic conceptions. However, clients who employ the theory of humoral imbalance may utilize allopathic facilities for treatment. For most clients, allopathy and Ayurveda have been assimilated within a general medical framework which focuses on the physiological functioning of the body. The use of allopathic therapeutic techniques is not perceived as challenging the Ayurvedically derived conceptual framework on which everyday, commonsense psychiatric understanding rests. To the client, the two subsystems are not perceived as conflicting and mutually exclusive, but as alternate strategies which address the same basic problem, the disorder of *māthāra golamāla* or head malfunctioning.

One of the striking features of the psychiatric domain is the paucity of Ayurvedic facilities in the midst of the predominance of a popular version of Ayurvedic theory. Why do Bengalis fail to patronize Ayurvedic facilities? Conversely, why do they seek out allopathic practitioners?

The institutionalization of medical care at the governmental level has had an important impact on the social position of both allopathic and Ayurvedic medicine. While the government had hoped to revive the practice of Ayurvedic medicine, it is also clear that,

> Yet as Ayurvedic schools were founded and their facilities improved, they appeared to become inferior versions of modern medical colleges....The reasons were clear enough: even the few graduates who became successful private practitioners would not enjoy the legal privileges of modern doctors, and in the state health services physicians trained in these schools were considered qualified only for positions with low pay and limited responsibility (Leslie 1974:100).

The privileged position granted allopathic practitioners has been important in establishing the greater prestige and availability of allopathic psychiatry (Leslie, 1980). It is therefore understandable that recent studies (Kapur, 1979; Srinivasa and Trivedi, 1982) report that allopathic medicine is most often the initial treatment preference for mentally disturbed patients. However, the legal and social status of allopathic medicine and its increased availability hardly compel clients to patronize allopathic facilities. Folk psychiatry, for instance, has resisted these pressures of modernization and the <u>ōjhā</u> have survived as sought-after psychiatric specialists. Thus, these factors do not fully explain the popularity of allopathy.

In order to understand the clients' willingness to initiate and maintain a relationship with allopathic practitioners, it is necessary to examine the relationship between clients and specialists in more detail. A psychiatric system, as a structural relationship between specialists and clients, depends on meaningful interaction between the two roles. Thus, the fact that clients are willing to initiate and maintain a therapeutic relationship with allopathic specialists must be because they view interaction with allopathic psychiatrists as meaningful. Though clients grant specialists considerable authority to define the situation for them, clients have the option to withdraw from the interaction. If clients perceive allopathy as being in opposition to their own medical knowledge, and perceive the specialists' behavior as a violation of their expectations regarding treatment, they can terminate the relationship. In actuality, however, clients do seek allopathic treatments and therefore must be interpreting the specialists' behavior as an attempt to cure the patients. Such an interpretation is possible because the theories and behavior of the specialists are at least marginally congruent with the clients' own conceptions.

While the psychiatrist uses the theoretical category "mental illness" and the client uses "head disturbance" (māthāra golamāla), the two concepts have phenotypical appearances or symptoms which overlap considerably. The major difference is that the psychiatrist's definition of "mental illness" is broader than the client's concept of māthāra golamāla. While many psychiatrists complain that Bengalis fail to seek treatment in less severe cases of disorder, the psychiatrist is likely to view the patient who is brought to the allopathic clinic with suspected māthāra golamāla as appropriate for psychiatric treatment. This congruence at the phenotypic level makes it difficult for either psychiatrist or client to realize that māthāra golamāla and "mental illness" are actually quite different theoretical entities.

Furthermore, both actors assume that "mental illness" m̄athāra golamāla is a medical problem, i.e., one involving the psycho-physiological processes of the patient. This minimal theoretical congruence means that phenomena that clients cite as relevant symptoms are also recognized by psychiatrists as relevant symptoms. Both physiological complaints such as headache, heart palpitations, sleeplessness, and loss of appetite, and psychological disturbances such as hostility, lethargy, and hallucinations, are regarded as psychiatric symptoms by both clients and specialists. If the client mentions these, the psychiatrist will affirm their importance. If the psychiatrist inquires about them, the client will recognize their significance as possible symptoms. Thus, while the suspected meaning of the symptoms may vary substantially, judgments as to their relevance are fairly congruent.

A similar situation exists with regard to etiology. The client's concept of "shock" tends to overlap with the psychiatrist's concept of stress. The psychiatrist is likely to acknowledge the importance of such events as the death of a loved one, failure in examinations, and inability to have children. While the dynamics by which events are etiologically linked to the patient's disorder vary tremendously, the procedure of taking a personal history conforms to the client's expectations of a specialist. The psychiatrist wants to know the very information that the client feels it is important to provide.

Finally, allopathic treatment is also consistent with the client's expectations. Medicine is almost invariably given, which is appropriate from the client's perspective. Clients also view hospitalization and electro-convulsive shock as reasonable. In fact, clients will often request electric shock treatments as a means to counteract the earlier "shock."

Within the interactional context of allopathic therapeutic procedures, these assumptions regarding symptoms, etiology, and treatment produce behavior on the part of both client and allopathic psychiatrist that can be "understood" by the other. Furthermore, the nature of their respective role expectations requires only a minimal set of shared assumptions, making it unlikely that the basic misunderstanding will be detected. By acknowledging the psychiatrist's expertise, the client does not expect that there will be a complete consensus between them. On the contrary, rather than challenging the assumptions of shared frames of reference, discrepancies reinforce the role relationship of medical practitioner and client. For example, if the client mentions a symptom -- such as burning sensations (Chakraborty, 1971) or sperm loss (Carstairs, 1956) -- which is irrelevant from within the allopathic framework, the psychiatrist translates it into psychiatric terminology (e.g., hypochondria or delusional material). Conversely, if the psychiatrist inquires about a symptom, such as a change in libido, that is irrelevant from the client's perspective, the client is likely to view the question as evidence of the psychiatrist's superior medical expertise. Thus, the unequal authority in the role relationship between client and psychiatrist necessitates only a certain minimal cognitive congruence in order for meaningful interaction to take place.

A second reason why the basic cognitive differences are not detected is the pragmatic, a-theoretical basis for the interaction. The purpose-at-hand, for both psychiatrist and client, is to cure the patient. Because the major concern is therapeutic, there need not be any discussion of fundamental cognitive orientation. The psychiatrist rarely discusses either diagnosis or etiology with the patient or accompanying relatives; nor are the latter likely to make such inquiries, since they might be construed as challenging the expertise of the psychiatrist. In the frequent cases of referral to psychiatrists from other allopathic doctors, the client may not even realize that the somatic symptoms have been redefined as a psychiatric disorder. In general, the client is satisfied if the specialist provides reasonable treatment and the psychiatrist is satisfied if the client follows instructions.

Thus, both the norms of the role relationship and a certain degree of shared conceptions enable clients and allopathic specialists to interact meaningfully. Since their own conceptual orientation derives from Ayurveda, clients are rarely confronted with the fact that Ayurveda and allopathy are quite different theoretical systems. For clients, Ayurveda and allopathy have become assimilated into a single psychiatric subsystem. It is only at this point that the greater prestige and availability of allopathy are likely to influence clients' treatment-seeking decisions.

Interaction between practitioner and client takes place within a low degree of cognitive congruence. This observation is especially significant in the light of the debate over the role of cognitive systems in health care system (Kunstadter, 1978). While I would agree with Kleinman (1980) that the client's explanatory model (i.e., the paradigm used to interpret a given instance of illness) shapes and organizes the treatment-seeking process, it is less clear how crucial it is that the practitioner and client share the same cognitive model. In the Bengali case, the norms of the role relationship between practitioner and client, namely the differential authority and the pragmatic therapeutic focus, enable clients and allopathic psychiatrists to interact meaningfully with only a minimal set of shared conceptions.[2]

Structural Pluralism

This discussion of Ayurveda and allopathy also highlights the importance of the concept of structural pluralism. Clients and practitioners view the entire medical system quite differently. On the one hand, interaction between client and allopathic psychiatrist is unlikely to disrupt the client's assumption that psychiatrists use the same paradigm of <u>māthāra golamāla</u> that they do. On the other hand, psychiatrists are very much aware of their divergence from Ayurvedic practitioners and view such divergence from the perspective of competitive ideological systems. Therefore, practitioner and client, the role positions within the psychiatric domain, have two distinct views of the structure of that domain. The point, however, is not simply that clients and specialists view the system differently. The point is that there <u>is</u> a competitive structure at the level of specialist relationships and that there <u>is</u> an assimilation structure at the level of client behavior. These two divergent structures represent the third type of pluralism, structural pluralism.

Structural pluralism refers to the contrasting structures which emerge from the psychiatric behavior of various actors. Recognition that there are divergent structures of the psychiatric domain raises the theoretical issue of the concept of "structure" itself. It is my argument that the social structure of an area of sociocultural experience must be conceived of as social praxis, as derived from the concrete behavior of specific individuals acting in particular social settings. Therefore, "objective structures of social activities are to be regarded as the situated practical accomplishments of the work through and by which the appearance-of-objective-structures is displayed and detected" (Zimmerman and Pollner 1970:103). Structure cannot be divorced from the behavior of actors as they interact within a given sociocultural setting.

This view of structure is based on Garfinkel's (1967) formulation of the reflexivity of social behavior. Summarizing Garfinkel's argument, Filmer states:

> Garfinkel is contending that what we take to be the objective features of social reality are objective only because we express them in objective terms....[Such objective features] are not necessarily intrinsic to the objects and events themselves, but are given to them by the manner in which they are described....[A]t the everyday level the process of explanation is synonymous with the construction of social reality, of social life itself. Thus, in accounting for their actions in a rational way, members are <u>making</u> those actions rational and thus making social life a coherent and comprehensible reality in a way that underlines the constructed nature of all reality (1972:212).

The essential reflexivity of social behavior means that structure emerges from the very social activities which are organized by that structure. Rather than postulating "social structure" and "social behavior" as two different orders of reality between which interrelationships must be specified, it is my position that the two must be treated as mutually constitutive of each other. Structure is then a social process, equivalent to the structuring behavior of social actors. Mehan develops this point in his study of the school setting, calling his approach "constitutive ethnography":

> ...the interactional work of participants structures the educational facts of these school settings....Constitutive ethnographers...put structures and structuring on an equal footing by showing how the social facts of the educational world emerge from structuring activities to become external and constraining... (1978: 59, 60).

From this point of view, a "pluralistic" structure exists only to the extent that actors behave in such a way that its existence is affirmed; i.e., so as to differentiate various subsystems as distinct entities. Even though the observer or researcher may conclude that the subsystems encompass conflicting and mutually exclusive theoretical bases, a psychiatric system is pluralistic only when the behavior of the actors themselves serve to distinguish between subsystems. With the concept of structural pluralism, I am postulating that there are two different kinds of behavior which serve to structure the psychiatric domain: the practitioners' behavior with regard to each other, and the clients' behavior with regard to seeking treatment.

Within the first category of social action, practitioners interact with each other in many ways which structure the psychiatric domain. For example, a psychoanalyst who uses Yogic exercises with his patients communicates certain things about the relationship between psychoanalysis and Yoga, and therefore is involved in structuring the psychiatric domain in a certain way. Similarly, the Ayurvedic practitioner who decries the use of electric shock is structuring a particular relationship between Ayurveda and allopathy. The practitioners' behavior structures the psychiatric domain to the extent that it serves to maintain or obscure, to enhance or minimize, the distinctions between the subsystems. Simply put, the psychiatric domain has a pluralistic institutional structure because the patterned interaction among the practitioners establishes and reinforces institutional boundaries. Similarly, the structural relationship between allopathy and Ayurveda at the institutional level is one of competition so long as practitioners of each system act toward each other as rivals.

But the structure of the psychiatric domain cannot be restricted to patterned behavior among psychiatric practitioners. Clients' behavior, and especially treatment-seeking strategies, also constitute the structure of the system. From this point of view, the psychiatric system is one of cognitive pluralism because clients make distinctions between the three conceptual paradigms to organize and justify treatment strategies. Similarly, Ayurveda and allopathy have become assimilated to the extent that client behavior does not distinguish between the two, i.e., at the point where a client takes a patient with _māthāra golamāla_ to an allopathic psychiatrist.

At times, the structure that emerges from the two kinds of behavior is the same. For example, the structural relationships of folk psychiatry are the same whether one examines the behavior of the folk healers or the behavior of the psychiatric clients. Both behave so as to affirm its particularistic position within the psychiatric domain. But the important point is that it cannot be assumed that the structure which emerges through the behavior of the practitioners will be congruent with that which is constituted by the clients' behavior. The structure of allopathy and Ayurveda is one of competition and one of assimilation, because both kinds of behavior -- relationships among practitioners and clients' treatment-seeking behavior -- structure the psychiatric domain. It is just such a situation which has been described as structural pluralism: plural structures which derive from differing structuring behavior.

This analysis of structural pluralism dictates that the researcher must be careful to specify clearly what behavior is being used as data in constructing an analysis of the medical or psychiatric domain. Failure to do so has led to the tendency to equate "the" structure with that which derives from the practitioners' behavior. If we identify a pluralistic structure as one incorporating several subsystems with distinctive professional ideologies and institutional facilities, we are only focusing on institutional pluralism and the role of the practitioner within the system. There are two pitfalls to such a procedure. On the one hand, the impact that the clients' behavior has on these same institutions is often neglected. The secure institutional position that allopathic psychiatry has within the psychiatric domain in Bengal is at least partially attributable to the fact that its use has become assimilated within the māthāra golamāla paradigm used by clients. On the other hand, clients' behavior may make little sense if we only view it in terms of the structures which derive from the practitioners' ideology and institutions. Clients' behavior has to be analyzed in terms of the cognitive system that clients themselves use to account for their behavior and to make it meaningful.

A more serious problem is the tendency to reify social structure, which then clouds its relationship to social behavior. As noted by ethnomethodologists (Zimmerman and Pollner, 1970; Phillipson, 1972), to account for social behavior in terms of social structural features is to adopt the "natural attitude of everyday life" in social research. Within the natural attitude, the social world is available as a "resource" for explanation. The "objective" reality of social structure is accepted as given and used to explain other social phenomena (e.g., why individuals behave the way they do). A recognition that social structure is an accomplishment of social praxis transforms structure into a "topic." The researcher is then sensitized to the need for examining structuring behavior, that by which structure is accomplished and objectified.[3] It is crucial to begin to reconceptualize pluralism in terms of the structuring behavior of social actors.

NOTES

1. Major works in the area of medical pluralism include Kleinman, 1980; Kleinman et al., 1978; Janzen, 1978; and Leslie, 1976b and 1980.

2. Horton (1967a, 1967b) discusses a similar situation, where interaction among traders from different cultures does not expose the cultural discrepancies between the two. Similarly, it would seem that psychodynamic therapies would require a higher degree of cognitive congruence, perhaps an additional reason for their restricted use in Bengal.

3. The present emphasis on behavior as structuring the system is not meant to deny the constraining effect of the structure which thereby emerges. Rather, that the structure is "objective," "external," and "constraining" is itself accomplished through social action.

For a similar kind of argument, see Weider's discussion of the "convict code" which characterizes the normative expectations governing the residents of a half-way house. He notes that: "'telling the code' created a social reality for persons who heard it...." (1974:159) Later he says:

> Thus, 'telling the code,' and any particular instance of formulating the code, <u>exhibits</u> rather than describes or explains, the order that members achieve through their practices of showing and telling each other that particularly encountered features are typical, regular, orderly, coherent, motivated out of onsideration for normative constraint, and the like (1974:171).

Part II

TWO THEORIES OF PĀGALĀMI

CHAPTER 5

Pagalami as Frustrated Desire

The internal structure of the psychiatric domain has been analyzed through an examination of the social roles of and relationship between client and specialist. But since the psychiatric domain also includes the patient, it is also necessary to analyze that role. One of the key characteristics of the patient role is that the patient is viewed as the embodiment of pāgalāmi. As that which provides substantiality and materiality to pāgalāmi, the patient represents the corporal expression of pāgalāmi. An indication of this aspect of the patient role is the tendency for others to treat the patient's behavior as symptoms. Whereas the psychiatrists view responses from the client as descriptions of the disorder, responses from the patient are seen as symptoms of the disorder.[1] In such instances, the social meaning of the patient's behavior is not established by reference to the interaction but by reference to pāgalāmi. The patient is treated not as a social actor but as the material representation of the disease entity.[2] Thus, from this perspective, an analysis of the role of the patient is at the same time an analysis of pāgalāmi, and thus will serve to locate the psychiatric domain within the larger context of Bengali culture.

To analyze pāgalāmi, it is necessary to delineate the moral meanings actors construct in the situated context of their behavior. When Bengalis identify a particular phenomenon (behavior, event, individual, etc.) as being *pāgalāmi*, they are communicating that certain moral meanings and a certain theory of the world apply to that phenomenon. They are saying that the phenomenon possesses the quality of *pāgalāmi* and therefore it becomes socially constituted as a particular kind of social object. The properties which are conferred upon the phenomenon through this labeling process comprise the concept and theory of *pāgalāmi*. Conversely, to analyze what *pāgalāmi* is, it is necessary to formulate that theory by establishing the properties which are asserted through the application of the label *pāgalāmi*.

Probably the most important characterization of *pāgalāmi* is that it is deviance. Deviance refers to a property conferred upon behavior which indicates that it is outside the cultural boundaries of the group (Erikson 1966:6ff). Thus, deviance stimulates a reaction that communicates that the behavior is judged as inappropriate, immoral, or otherwise not in accordance with the normative expectations which apply in that particular context. One such deviance-generating response is a corrective or therapeutic one. From this perspective, the client-specialist relationship is important because it confers this fundamental attribute of deviance on *pāgalāmi*. The evaluation that a particular sociopsychological event is an instance of *pāgalāmi* entails treatment-seeking behavior and a therapeutic response on the part of significant others.

To formulate the theory of *pāgalāmi*, we must examine the ways in which *pāgalāmi* is deviance, the ways in which *pāgalāmi* deviates from the normative expectations which Bengalis have of each other. If "social groups create deviance by making the rules whose infraction constitutes deviance" (Becker 1963:9), then pāgalāmi is best defined by locating the rules which generate pāgalāmi, the boundaries which pāgalāmi transgresses. As Erikson (1966) has noted, interaction surrounding deviance communicates to the members of a community where the group's normative boundaries lie, and thus locates the group's cultural space. To delimit a particular deviant category such as pāgalāmi is a means by which that cultural territory can be identified. Examining pāgalāmi as deviance establishes the broader cultural relevance of the psychiatric domain as a border area that locates the Bengali cultural space within. I will identify two aspects of the theory of pāgalāmi: pāgalāmi as frustrated desire and pāgalāmi as entropy. In each case, pāgalāmi depends on concepts of human nature and establishes the normative relationship between human beings and the surrounding environment.

Pāgalāmi and Frustration

As previously noted, "shock" is identified as a major etiological factor involved in māthāra golamāla [head malfunctioning]. In addition to the case histories cited earlier, non-client Bengalis who were asked why people become pāgala also used the concept of "shock." Both the English word "shock" and the Bengali term āghāta [a heavy blow, either mental or physical] were used frequently. Other common words were śoka [mourning, grief], duḥkha [sorrow], cintā [worry], abhāva [insufficiency], and mānasika dvanda [mental conflict]. Some of the responses I obtained were:

> If one worries, because of money or illness, one becomes pāgala. If a shock (āghata) strikes the head hard, then one will become pāgala.
>
> Because of poverty. If one fails when studies are good, one will become pagala. If "shock" is received, one will become pāgala....If the head becomes hot from sorrow (duhkha), it happens....Many become pāgala from "love affairs."
>
> If one worries a lot about some little thing..., if one thinks intensely about it, māthāra golamāla can happen. If there is some "deficiency," māthāra golamāla happens. If he wants something but can't get it.

The terms people used, and the examples provided to illustrate them, all point to frustration as a key factor. Frustration might be caused by economic worries, academic failure, lack of career advancement, or unrequited love. Several respondents made general statements about failure to obtain some deeply desired goal:

> If one doesn't get something wanted wholeheartedly, one becomes pāgala -- be it consciously desired or unconsciously.
>
> Someone wants something, "wants it desperately," but didn't get it.
>
> Perhaps in his mind, he wanted something, but didn't get it. If a man wants something a lot but doesn't get it, he becomes unhappy (aśānti), the mind breaks (mana bheṅge pare) and he becomes pāgala.

The most extreme example of such frustration and the one most frequently cited was śoka, intense grief and longing due to the death of a loved one:

> It happens from "shock"; if the only child dies.
>
> If one receives a lot of sadness (duḥkha), one will become pāgala. When the sadness crosses the limits of endurance, then one will become pāgala.

Thus, the primary attribute of "shock" is an emotional response to an intensely frustrating situation. Some obstacle puts the desired outcome beyond one's control, thus rendering ineffectual one's own efforts to obtain it. In such a situation, the individual's wants, needs, and desires go unfulfilled. The implicit image seems to be the almost physical accumulation of emotion and thus the generation of intense pressure on the brain.

This analysis is complemented by the belief that pāgalāmi can be cured if the desires of the individual are satisfied. For an unmarried patient, marriage is often recommended as a way to meet the patient's needs for both affection and sex. In an article in the Bengali newspaper Ananda Bazar Patrika, the reporter comments that one patient "might fully recover if she can get her boyfriend back." Similarly, having a baby is thought to cure mental illness in women. One infertile patient told me that all her problems and compulsive behavior would disappear as soon as she got pregnant. To regain mental health, the source of the patient's worries and frustration must be removed. Perhaps this view of the mentally ill as experiencing extreme frustration is also responsible for the gentleness with which family members often treat patients.

The concept of "shock" points to the belief that excessive desire can have destructive consequences for the individual. The emphasis is on the harmful role of frustration, when desires cannot be gratified. This theme is found in classical Sanskrit literature, is echoed throughout other areas of Bengali culture, and is also incorporated into the theories of G.S. Bose, the founder of a Bengali version of psychoanalysis.

Even as early as the Upanisads, the idea is introduced that passion inhibits self-realization and that salvation (liberation, mokṣa) is dependent on a state of non-attachment. Thus, self-realization can occur only "when all the desires that dwell within the human heart are cast away...when all the knots that fetter the heart are cut asunder" (from the Katha Upanisad, quoted in Murphy and Murphy 1968:59). The liberated man has abandoned his worldly attachments and is free from desire or passion. Passion, as the motivational force which connects the individual to the objects of the environment, causes man's attachment to the phenomenal world, thereby impeding spiritual release.

In the Bhagavad Gita, passion is linked with rajas [energy, activity], one of the three guṇa or attributes. Action characterized by the attribute sattva involves the performance of dharma [duty] and is contrasted with rajas involving the expression of kāma [passion]. In contrast with the ideal of the Upanisads, where spiritual salvation is attained through withdrawal from the phenomenal world, the Gita teaches a philosophy of action, but action guided by duty. As De Bary (1958:276) notes, "action, as such, is not detrimental to one's attainment of his spiritual goal. It is only one's attachment to the fruits of action" that prevents liberation. Though action in the world is permitted, salvation is still associated with the control of passion and the senses so as to sever the self's attachment to the world. The description of the self-realized individual is a portrayal of one whose desires have been extinguished:

> He is known as one with equipoise...when he eschews all overmuch desire and learns to be satisfied with himself. Difficulties disturb him not and pleasures fail to tempt him; freed from longing, dread and hate, he is a sage with steady mind. His heart is settled in nothing, meeting good or evil he is neither happy nor sad. His senses are withdrawn, like the limbs of a turtle and his mind is steady. Objects of lust, unfed, disappear....Senses indeed are naughty and snatch the mind away. The wise one controls them all...for when they are controlled, mind can be steady. Brooding over objects of enjoyment, one gets fixed on them; being fixed he craves for them. Craving (unfulfilled) leads to anger, and anger to confusion, confusion makes for unreasonableness and that results in madness, which is the road to destruction. Bereft of love and hate, senses bridled by the self, the individual obtains calmness. In calmness so all cares and worries find their end; calmness helps the mind settle....When mind yields to the whims of senses, it is led hopelessly astray, like a boat on water wafted by the gale (<u>Bhagavad</u> <u>Gita</u> 2.55-71; quoted in Rao 1962: 179-80).

This theme of the negative and destructive consequences of passion is particularly highlighted in Yoga. By means of Yogic disciplinary exercises, the individual can achieve "complete liberation from the bonds of conditioned existence" (Jacobs 1961:90). Such liberation is attained through control of the senses and of passion. It is especially interesting that attempts have been made to establish the relevance of Yoga for the treatment of mental disturbances (Coster, 1934; Deshmukh, 1972; Goyeche, 1972; Joshi, 1964; Vahia, 1969; Vahia et al., 1966, 1972, 1973a, and 1973b; Brar, 1970; Masson, 1974; Pal, 1971; and Jacobs, 1961).

Vahia has attempted to formulate an explicit therapy based upon Yogic principles. He begins by noting that an individual's equilibrium can be disrupted by "disturbing thoughts...associated with Raga [emotional attachment to appealing objects] or Dvesha [hatred or jealousy towards ...objects...]" (1969:7). As the six major factors which "disrupt the harmony," Vahia lists kama [desire, lust], krodha [anger], lobha [greed], moha [delusion, infatuation], mada [exaggerated self-concept], and matsara [jealousy].* The patient's "concentration" is disrupted by such thoughts, and thus Vahia argues that "it [is] not so much the environmental stress, but his [i.e., the patient's] reaction to it that [is] of primary importance" (1969:7). Furthermore, it is the patient's egocentricity or the "desire to maintain his self-esteem" which is the underlying cause of all these factors.

Vahia argues that the goal of therapy is to help the patient become less affected by such disturbing thoughts. The first step is to help the patient

> understand in a detached and objective manner the various factors that produce positive feelings like love and affection and negative feelings like anger and fear, which all disturb his mind....He would now appreciate that his preoccupation with the maintenance of self-esteem was primarily responsible for his inadequate adjustment" (1969:9, 10).

By decreasing the importance of his egoistic self-esteem, the patient will be able to eliminate the disturbing thoughts, to concentrate on objective goals, and

---

*His spelling and English glosses.

to become independent of environmental responses to his behavior which would otherwise cause stress and anxiety.

This belief in the destructive potential of passion is also evident in contemporary ethnographic data. An example is the common somatic complaint of extreme weakness and lethargy attributed to the loss of semen (Carstairs, 1956; Bagadia, 1973; Obeyesekere, 1976). Semen is one of the seven dhātu [body substances] of Ayurvedic theory. It is generally believed that a man has a fixed amount of semen. Not only is this reserve reduced during ejaculation, but semen can "leak" and "curdle." Since semen is considered the main source of a man's energy and power, any contamination or loss of semen is identified with a loss of strength. On the basis of Rajasthani data, Carstairs suggests that the cultural ideal, complete restraint from sexual activity, is generally compromised by subordinating sexuality to the services of dharma or the duty to satisfy one's wife and to have children. Furthermore, he and Brar (1970) both note that the conservation of semen is associated with one's ability to achieve liberation. Since semen provides the energizing force of the individual, preserving and channelling it facilitates self-realization and final liberation. This conceptualization is a more concretized version of the Sanskritic belief that salvation requires the control of passion.

In other contemporary cultural patterns, this attitude toward desire is evident in certain Bengali child-rearing practices. Western observers often comment that the Indian child is "spoiled." Indeed, it does appear that the major responsibility of other family members is to gratify the child's every whim (see Kakar, 1978; Carstairs, 1957; Spratt, 1966). A Bengali baby is seldom allowed to cry for long, at least without repeated efforts at soothing him/her. "Demand" nursing is the normal pattern, and weaning is not only slow and gradual but often delayed well into the second or even third year. Toilet training is accomplished with a minimum of harshness. As Surya (1969: 388) has commented, "A child rarely is exposed to the need to wait for anything or to stand any frustration for long. Any educative frustration of a child attempted by one member of the family is soon mollified by the over-protective attention of another." The most basic child-rearing rule appears to be: minimize frustration by gratifying all desires. An example of this principle involves the toys I had brought for my two infant nieces. Because the babies kept putting them in their mouths, the toys were quickly set out of their reach. My offer to teach them not to do so was simply ignored. Presumably, such restrictions would have produced a frustrating situation, and thus the best strategy was to remove the temptation. Overt conflict through direct commands or prohibitions was carefully avoided.

The two major exceptions to this generalization, the feeding and studies situations, simply reinforce this conclusion. From an early age, all three of the bottle-fed babies with whom I was familiar were forcibly fed with a spoon, in spite of protesting cries. However, such coercion was definitely a last resort; mothers and other family members might spend a full hour cajoling the child to eat, using distractions, bribes, and threats. Thus, while coercion was used, there was a tacit recognition that it was only acceptable given the essential nature of eating. The second exception was the conflict over studies. It was assumed that school children had to be made to study and, again, family members spent considerable time helping with homework or just nagging children to finish their studies. Again, force aroused anxiety and was justified by the crucial importance of doing well in school. Thus, these exceptions only referred to the child's most basic obligations -- to grow healthy and to learn.

One of the rationales behind such gratification of the child is the need to encourage the child's even temperament (<u>ṭhāṇḍā</u> <u>mejāja</u>). Deprivation causes frustration and anger and thus predisposes the child to a greater likelihood of becoming frustrated and angry again. A vicious circle sets in. On the one hand, the child is believed to have little tolerance for frustration; on the other, early deprivation can have a lasting effect on the personality by making the child "hot-tempered" (<u>garama</u> <u>mejāja</u>). "Spoiling" the child precludes any frustration and thus preserves his/her emotional stability.[3]

Another example of belief in the necessity to satisfy desires is the <u>sādha</u> ritual. This ritual is performed after the seventh month of pregnancy and before the birth of the child. The primary aim of the occasion is to ensure that the pregnant woman has all her wishes fulfilled. Indeed, <u>sādha</u> means "desire" and is used in colloquial Bengali to indicate an intense longing or craving. The <u>sādha</u> ceremony involves a feast at which guests present the woman with saris and sweets, both luxuries for all but the wealthy. Interestingly, one Westernized Bengali woman who had dispensed with the traditional <u>sādha</u> told me that her <u>sādha</u> consisted of a dinner at a Chinese restaurant because she had been craving Chinese food. Specific food cravings are expected during pregnancy and, independent of the <u>sādha</u>, attempts are usually made to provide the desired foods. The rationale behind this practice is that unfulfilled desires can be injurious to both mother and child: *sādha* ensures an easy delivery and a healthy, happy (*ṭhāṇḍā mejāja*) baby.

In addition to *māthāra golamāla* and the concept of "shock," the other two paradigms of *pāgalāmi* also involve frustrated desire. A *bhūta* [ghost] is a disembodied self which has not obtained release so that it can proceed to the next life. Persons who die through *apaghāta-mṛityu* [unnatural death], that is, those who die "before their time," are particularly likely to become *bhūta*. *Bhūta*, then, are the selves of persons whose death does not entail their detachment from the world of the living, which is especially the case of persons who die before they are able to live out their lives in full. This residual attachment to the world of the living is apt to occur if the individual dies without having satisfied important passions. An unmarried man (i.e., one who has had no sexual experiences) and a childless woman are prime candidates for becoming *bhūta*. It is also important to link this conception of the *bhūta* with the two instances noted above where every effort is made to satisfy desires, for childhood and pregnancy are two times when the individual is especially vulnerable and the possibility of an untimely death the greatest. Thus, it would seem that gratification of all wants would be an attempt to enhance the likelihood of release in the event of death and, conversely, to preclude the possibility of the self becoming a *bhūta*.

Sorcery (*tuka*) also represents an example of the destructive consequences of frustrated desire. For example, there is a common belief that the childless woman's longing for a child may motivate her to bewitch another's child. Her desires are so strong that any indication of her attraction to a child arouses the fear that she may unintentionally cast an "evil eye" on the child. Generally, tuka is the result of envy and jealousy of others who possess desirable qualities lacking in oneself. The mother of an unsuccessful student might be suspected of performing tuka on her son's more intelligent classmates, or a jilted lover of bewitching the husband of his former lover. As noted, the new bride is frequently the object of envy by those in her new household. Thus, the basic cause of sorcery is deprivation and the frustration of one's desires.

The Work of G.S. Bose

Since the theme of the negative effects of frustration is reminiscent of Freud's theories of repression, anxiety, and mental disorder, it is not surprising to find that psychoanalytic theory has attracted considerable attention in Bengal. The Indian Psychoanalytic Society has its national headquarters in Calcutta and, in 1975, 14 of India's 39 trained analysts resided there. It has established an inpatient facility (Lumbini Park Mental Hospital), an outpatient clinic (G.S. Bose Clinic) and two journals (Samiksha and Citta). The English-language journal Samiksha began publication in 1947, three years before the Indian Psychiatric Association began publishing its journal. The Indian Psychoanalytic Institute has been training analysts since 1930, whereas Calcutta University established the Diploma of Psychological Medicine only in 1959.

The prestige of psychoanalysis in Bengal can be attributed to the dynamic and charismatic personality of

Girindrasekhar Bose. Born in 1887, Bose received degrees in both medicine and psychology. In 1929, he became the Head of the Department of Psychology at Calcutta University and remained in that position for 20 years. It appears that Bose may have become familiar with Freud's work as early as 1909, and in 1921, he and Freud began a correspondence that was to last for 16 years (Ramana, 1964).[4] While Bose's doctoral thesis, Concept of Repression, was written in 1920, before he had the benefit of consulting Freud's work in detail, he viewed his own work as "an extension and an amplification of the existing psychoanalytic theories and also an effort at their unification" (Bose 1966:86-7).

The main features of Bose's view are clear in his "theory of opposite wish." In this theory, Bose (1966:71) postulates that every wish is "a peculiar psychic process conscious or unconscious which precedes or accompanies the tendency of the organism in its effort to change the environment so as to have an adjustment different from the existing one." Bose argues that in order to formulate a wish, the individual must "have some sort of appreciation of the object." This appreciation of and identification with the object, required in order to formulate a wish at all, necessitates that the individual must formulate the opposite wish at the same time. "Every wish that arises in consciousness is accompanied by its opposite which remains in the unconscious" (1966:82). Thus, an active wish is accompanied by a passive wish. The wish to strike is accompanied by the wish to be struck; the wish to love triggers the wish to be loved. For unless what is implied by being struck or being loved is understood through identification, the individual cannot desire to strike or to love. Wishes, then, always exist as opposing pairs.

Since both wishes cannot be satisfied simultaneously, one of them will become repressed.

Thus, Bose's term "wish" is comparable to Freud's "id." While both of these are seen as motivational and energizing factors of the personality, there are two crucial differences. First, wish, as opposed to the id, is not instinctual; the content varies depending on the state of the individual and the particular relation to the environment. That wishes occur as an opposing pair is a logical "necessity," not a physiological one. Second, the motivational force of the wish is directed towards instrumental action, that is, toward achieving a changed adaptation to the environment. While it is certainly clear that the satisfaction of id drives also requires environmental response, the focus is more expressive than instrumental.

In Bose's work, repression seems to be more dependent on environmental frustration of wishes than is Freud's concept of repression. Bose (1966:85) argues that "repeated compulsory satisfaction of one of the wishes of a pair to the neglect of the other owing to one-sided environmental influences is responsible for bringing about a repression of the latter wish." For Freud, suppression only becomes repression when the superego introjects the moral principles of the surrounding society, thus prohibiting even conscious awareness of id desires. Bose, however, saw the superego as the product of repression ("the opposite counterparts of the oedipus tendencies") and believed that his theory "will render the conception of super-ego unnecessary" (1966:90). Freudian theory postulates a dynamic tension and conflict between the individual and the society which is lacking in Bose's work. By eliminating the superego as prior to repression and by linking the opposite wishes logically, Bose views the source of repression as residing either within the contradictory nature of wishes or within the environment.

From the previous discussion, it is clear that the psychological assumptions from Bose's cultural environment influenced his work. It would even seem that Bose may have found Freud's work congenial because it tended to reflect psychological conceptions already prevalent in Bengali culture. Bose's work could be said to represent a Freudian interpretation of themes that are recurrent both in the classical Sanskritic literature and in the cultural milieu of his own society. The id, as the motivational energy, is already recognizably similar to kāma and rajas. By transforming the Freudian id into "wish," Bose is able to assimilate conceptions from his own cultural heritage. First, wish becomes the instrumental means of relating to the environment. Second, with the theory of opposite wish, Bose asserts the destructive potential of wish. In both Hindu philosophy and Bose's psychoanalysis, it is the nature of man's desires which obstruct self-realization. From this perspective, Bose's work, as a study of "wish," follows in the tradition of inquiring into the nature of passion.

Desire in Bengali Ethnopsychology

This survey of the role of passion in Bengali ethnopsychology reveals the fundamental belief in the destructive capabilities of desire and passion. Two themes can be extracted. On the one hand, ethnographic evidence indicates that unsatisfied desires are believed to produce deleterious results and that a prerequisite for physical and psychological health is the gratification of desire. On the other hand, following the Sanskritic tradition, passion hinders liberation, and thus a prerequisite of salvation is freedom from passion. On first inspection, the themes appear contradictory. While the first argues for the expression and fulfillment of desires, the second encourages the subjugation of desire and its elimination as a prelude to final release. However, the two themes can be integrated into a common framework.

The ideal state of passionlessness does not refer to the suppression of desire but rather to the emancipation from desire. Thus, freedom from passion and the satisfaction of passion are both in opposition to a state of thwarted desire. Conversely, frustration can be avoided either by the satisfaction of desires or by the elimination of desire altogether. In this sense, the two themes simply provide two different alternatives to a culturally recognized malignant state. To use a metaphor which is particularly apt in the Indian context, where passion is identified with heat, a state of "firelessness" can be achieved by extinguishing the fire (i.e., gratification) or by controlling the conditions which cause a fire (i.e., self-control, detachment).

Each of the two alternatives is appropriate for certain people in certain situations according to their svadharma, their own specific moral code of conduct. The task of learning to be free of passion is viewed as a gradual process. According to Hindu thought, the life cycle of the individual can be divided into four āśrama [stages]: apprenticeship, householder, hermit, and sage. While the earlier stages prepare the individual for release, it is only in the last stage that the individual is expected to gain control over his desires as a means to attain moksa. Thus, the Sanskrit doctrine of freedom from passion is applicable only to the individual within the last stage of life. Furthermore, as an intermediary stage on the way to ultimate emancipation, the fulfillment of desire is permitted and may actually facilitate ultimate renunciation. The implication is that attachment to the world may be strengthened when desires are frustrated.

Moreover, the determination of one's proper svadharma [personal duty] is not only dependent on one's āśrama, but is also relative to one's other attributes (Kakar, 1968). Thus, the dharma of a child or a woman is considered different from that of a man in any of the stages of life. Childhood is not included in the āśrama, and apprenticeship begins with a boy's "second birth" at the time of receiving the sacred thread at age 12 or 13. Until that time, the child does not possess the intellect or other attributes required to begin the road to salvation. Similarly, the stages of life are not relevant to women. By virtue of the attributes associated with femininity, "their true function was marriage and the care of their menfolk and children" (Basham 1959:178). It would appear that the very nature of women and children negates the expectation to refrain from the expression and satisfaction of passion. Indeed, it is just in the case of women and children that the cultural injunction on frustration of desires is most evident.

Thus, the two themes can be integrated by recognizing that the philosophico-religious directive to be free from passion is specific for a man at the stage of renunciation. For others, their inherent attributes and the undeveloped state of their spirituality precludes emancipation from passion. Desire and its expression, if not valued, are at least to be expected. And, since such persons are not able to control their passions, it is best

FIGURE 2

Desire in Bengali Ethnopsychology

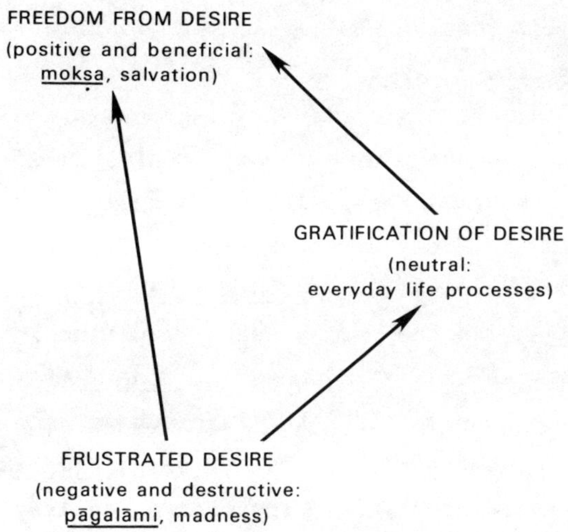

that they be gratified. Figure 2 illustrates this relationship between the three states of desire. As alternatives to a negative and destructive state of frustrated desire, both gratification of desire and freedom from desire are acceptable. Passionlessness is the preferred alternative, but it is unattainable for children, women, and the spiritually immature. Nonetheless, the gratification of desire is advantageous in the face of the detrimental consequences of unfulfilled passion. Within this scheme, the position of pāgalāmi as deviance is clear. It is the direct result of frustrated desire -- whether the "shock" of māthāra golamāla, the envy which causes tuka, or the early death resulting in bhūta bhara [ghost possession]. Madness or pāgalāmi becomes the concrete expression of the destructive and pernicious effects of frustrated desire. Thus pāgalāmi, as the deviance associated with frustrated desire, stands in juxtaposition to the everyday, neutral state of the satisfaction of desire and testifies to the harmful effects of frustrated desire. As a malignant state of human existance, pāgalāmi is a category of deviance which informs Bengalis of a basic human need -- the need to avoid frustration and to obtain the satisfaction of one's wants and desires.

Furthermore, pāgalāmi testifies to the vulnerability of human beings in the face of the potent nature of their desires. So long as individuals rely on the gratification of passion to protect them from the destructive potential of their own emotions, they are dependent on the whims of an environment which can prevent such gratification. Thus, pāgalāmi is a continual possibility; again, the Gita says that "craving (unfulfilled) leads to anger, and anger to confusion; confusion makes for unreasonableness and that results in madness, which is the road to destruction." It is in this sense that pāgalāmi represents an antithetical state from which the very meaning of salvation (mokṣa) is derived. By highlighting the very tentative and precarious relationship between human beings and their existential situation, pāgalāmi also indicates the solution to that human dilemma. To be mad is to be overwhelmed by one's emotions; to have attained salvation is to be released not only fron one's desires but also from the vulnerability of depending on environmental gratification of desires.

NOTES

1. Both the cognitive content and the expressive characteristics of the patient's talk may be treated as symptoms. The clearest example of the former is when the patient's fears about others' ill will are viewed as delusions rather than as a description of an actual social situation. Some excerpts from the psychiatrist's notes illustrate how the expressive features might be treated as symptoms: "voluble, talking away -- in grandiose fashion -- heavy religious colouring"; "somewhat dramatic and play acting. But also perplexed"; "patient talks freely but in disgruntled manner, detached from reality. Complains in a querulous tone about family member -- about being dominated."

2. I will not be examining the patient qua actor. However, one of the characteristics of that aspect of the patient role is often a denial of the patient as a fully competent social actor. It should also be noted that patients other than mental patients are often treated as embodying the particular disease. The recent critique that medicine in the West ignores the "whole person" is in response to the emphasis on the role of the patient qua disease entity.

3. At the same time, Bengalis often deliberately defer gratification, presumably to build up a tolerance for deprivation. If a child is given candy or other treats, an adult will almost inevitably entreat the child to give it away. A young child usually simply refuses (with the adult laughing in response), but the older child who does offer to give up the treat is told to go ahead and keep it. Teasing children that some promised reward won't be forthcoming is also common.

4. The Bose-Freud correspondence is reprinted in its entirety in the Indian Psychoanalytic Society journal Samiksha 10:2 and 10:3 (1956) and in Ramana, 1964. Some letters are obviously missing, since references are made to letters which are not included. In 1963, Freud's original letters, plus copies of Bose's, were deposited at the Sigmund Freud Archives, Vienna.

Freud's response to Bose is interesting. Over the 16 years during which they corresponded, he wrote 13 letters to the Indian psychoanalyst. While most are brief and non-substantive, four include Freud's evaluation of Bose's work. In his first letter, dated 1921, Freud wrote that he is "glad to testify [as to] the correctness of its [i.e., Bose's work, Concept of Repression] principal view and the good sense appearing in it." A year later, he wrote a preface to Concept of Repression acknowledging Bose's contribution to psychoanalysis. In 1929, Freud again commented on Bose's work: "it made a great impression on me. In fact, I am not convinced by your arguments. Your theory of the opposite wish appears to me to stress rather a formal element than a dynamic factor" (Ramana 1964:125). Shortly thereafter, Freud again wrote to Bose, saying that "the theory of opposite wishes strikes me as something less dynamical than morphological....It appears to me flat so to say, it seems to lack a third dimension. I don't think it is able to explain anxiety or the phenomenon of repression" (1964:130).

CHAPTER 6

Pāgalāmi as Entropy

The three basic psychiatric categories of bhūta bhara, tuka, and māthāra golamāla are related to each other because all three result in certain kinds of overt, observable behavior or symptomology which can be described as pāgalāmi. It is this conceptual fusion which dictates that the three are included within the psychiatric domain. One of the implications of examining pāgalāmi as deviance is the assumption that it is not merely linguistic or conceptual accident that these quite disparate phenomena fall within the psychiatric domain. The assumption postulates that it is these similarities which constitute pāgalāmi and the psychiatric domain as a distinct area of experience for Bengali actors. Therefore, it becomes pertinent to ask why the three genotypes should be included within the psychiatric domain, and to investigate the attributes they share. The fruitfulness of this approach is clear from the previous chapter: pāgalāmi as deviance represents the results of and thereby establishes the deleterious effects of frustrated desire. The three genotypes share an additional similarity, one which enables a clearer view of the psychiatric domain in Bengal.

Pāgalāmi and Boundary Maintenance

As noted in Chapter 2, Bengalis make a distinction between phenotypic and genotypic pāgalāmi. From this perspective, _bhara_ and _tuka_ can be juxtaposed to _māthāra golamāla_: _bhara_ and _tuka_ reflect a kind of pseudo-_pāgalāmi_, in the sense that they are not genotypic _pāgalāmi_. As such, they are things that happen to individuals, rather than something one becomes. Both involve an external agent -- whether a sorcerer's spell or possession by a ghost -- having an effect on the individual. In contrast, _māthāra golamāla_ seems to refer to an internal process resulting from an excess of heat and the ensuing humoral imbalance. However, to conceive of _māthāra golamāla_ as exclusively internal is to neglect a very fundamental aspect in the Bengali conceptualization of the individual. Since the individual is not an isolated, self-contained unit (Marriott, 1976; Marriott and Inden, 1976), the "internal" processes of humoral equilibrium or disequilibrium also imply a dynamic relationship between the individual and the environment.

Furthermore, to conceive of _māthāra golamāla_ as involving exclusively internal processes is to neglect the role of "shock" as the key etiological factor. The frustration which produces "shock" results from the occurrence (or non-occurrence) of some external, environmental event so that the individual is left without the means to satisfy certain desires and ambitions. "Shock" is a relational concept: a disjunction in the relationship between individual and environment wherein the environment frustrates desires.

From this point of view, _māthāra golamāla_ can also be conceptualized as the result of an outside agent, an environmental event such as _bhara_ or _tuka_ which has consequences for the individual. In all three cases, *pāgalāmi* involves a penetration of the individual by some outside agent. "Shock," *bhara*, and *tuka* all share a basic quality of intrusiveness; since intrusiveness implies a distinction between the outside and the inside, between the external and the internal, it also implies the existence of boundaries which separate the two spheres. *Pāgalāmi*, then, is a phenomenon which involves the disintegration of the boundaries separating outside and inside and, thus, a violation of the integrity of the individual. *Pāgalāmi* results from an implosive process wherein the outside intrudes upon the individual and obliterates the boundaries which maintain the distinctiveness of the individual. It is, in this sense, an entropic, order-reducing process because it entails the disintegration of the boundaries between distinctive units -- the individual and the environment.

This view of *pāgalāmi* is supported by the stereotypic view of the madman. When interviewing non-client Bengalis, I asked respondents to tell me of any mad persons they knew. Since many, especially the residents of the All Bengal Women's Union Home for Women, were unable to provide actual case histories, they often mentioned that they had seen mad people on the streets. These descriptions produced stereotypic answers on how a mad person behaves and provided crucial information for understanding the meaning of *pāgalāmi* as a category of deviance. Stereotypes provide the conceptual outlines of the social identity assumed after application of the deviant label. They are a clear statement of the social identity of the deviant "madman," unaffected by the influences of particular facts and experiences.[1]

Perhaps the most concise version of this stereotype is the response that "madmen don't do or say what ordinary people do and say." Some other descriptions are as follows:

> They roam here and there. They chase people. They roam about naked.
>
> Madmen behave according to their whim (<u>kheyāla</u> <u>khuśī</u> <u>mata</u>). They catch and beat everyone. They eat everything.
>
> I see a lot of madmen living on the street. According to their own inclination (<u>āpana</u> <u>mane</u>), they roam about, laugh, talk.
>
> They stay naked. They eat everything. They speak nonsense (<u>bak</u>-<u>bak</u> <u>bale</u>). This kind of madman I have seen.

Specifically, all respondents noted one or more of the following as characteristic of the madman: 1) has no home, lives on the street; 2) eats anything; 3) doesn't bathe; 4) is naked; 5) does whatever he wishes; 6) speaks jibberish. At the most elemental level, the Bengali view makes the madman a-cultural. Each of the characteristics of the madman is the inverse of some important aspect of Bengali culture: residence, consumption of food, bathing, clothing, rule-adherence, and language. Thus, the madman lives outside the cultural regulations which guide the behavior of Bengali everyday life.

What is significant about the image of the madman is that the stereotypic behaviors are not merely cultural violations, but violations of the very norms which seem to preserve, for Bengalis, a sense of the individual's own identity. For example, one's residence is highly identity-confirming. Most importantly, the individual resides with his/her family; thus one's <u>bāṛī</u> [house] establishes a group of kin-related persons whose relationship with the individual is crucial for one's sense of identity. It is common, for example, for a woman to identify herself as a *bāṛīra bau* or "wife of the house" to indicate that she is married to one of the male consanguine relatives who share the house. Furthermore, the location of that house, whether in the ancestral village or the current Calcutta neighborhood, is a key identifying fact. One of the more important things to know about a person (and consequently a frequent question among new acquaintances) is where one's house is located. For the madman to live in the streets and to roam about indicates that he has no *bāṛī*. He is, therefore, deprived of the identity which residence confers, both identity-defining kin relationships and a social status within the general community. To have no home is to be an outsider in a very fundamental way.

Similarly, one's own personal duty or moral code is clearly indicative of personal identity. Each individual has a personal code of conduct, *svadharma*, which defines one's moral obligations and thus the actions which must be performed. This personal moral code is dependent upon a variety of personal characteristics, locating a person as a member of several different groups of categories. As Inden and Nicholas (1977:xiv) point out, "each genus is defined by its particular substance (*dhātu*) and code (*dharma*) which are thought to be inseparable from one another." Because one's code for conduct is always embedded within one's substance, one's personal *dharma* involves not merely what one ought to do, but also what one is. *Dharma* is certainly a normative concept, but it also refers to one's basic nature. "In Bengali culture, there is a single order of beings, an order that in Western terms is both natural and moral, both material and spiritual" (1977:xiv). From this perspective, the fact that the madman does whatever he wishes and acts according to whim is an indication that he has no personal code of conduct, no dharma, and hence, in a significant sense, no identity at all.

In this regard, food habits become critical. Food regulations within Bengali culture are ubiquitous. They are established for various social statuses (e.g., the widow) and ritual occasions, as well as with regard to relationships among people (e.g., who can eat with whom). The sharing of food is particularly significant within the context of the family: jñāti kin (roughly, blood relatives) are identified as those who "share the same body" (Inden and Nicholas 1977:13). Further, "the sharing of food...most clearly and concretely expresses and sustains the shared body relationships of the persons of the same [family]..." (1977:18). To share food is to share the substances which will be transformed into the shared body of the family. Furthermore, because moral codes are "embodied" within substances, sharing food comes to signify the additional feature of a shared code for conduct. Thus, food regulations signify social relational solidarities which have crucial significance for personal identity. Again, the madman, by not adhering to these regulations, is dispossessed of these identity-confirming relationships.

The stereotypic madman, violating the norms of residence, of dharma, and of food consumption, loses the distinctiveness which sets him apart as an individual. With no home, no moral code, and no restrictions on food consumption, he forfeits the cultural means by which to ensure the preservation of his individual identity. But not only do these norms provide the individual with a sense of social and personal identity, they also regulate the individual's interactions with the environment. Place of residence signifies location within the environment, and food consumption involves the internalization of external, environmental objects. One's actions, one's dharma, are the means by which the individual relates to and acts upon the environment. Behaving indiscriminately, the madman fails to regulate his interaction with the environment in terms of dharma or duty, bāṛī or home, and khāoyā or eating. Without this careful regulation of behavior, residence, and food consumption, the boundaries which sustain the individual's differentiation from the surrounding environment, and thus his own distinctiveness and identity within that environment, disintegrate. The fact that a madman lives anywhere, eats everything, and does anything means that he is deprived of any personal identity beyond his madness.

In this context, it is also instructive to examine the curing procedures of the two temples, Tirole and Chakrapur. At both, the ritual cure of pāgalāmi involves four basic components: bathing, wearing the bālā [bangle], observing food restrictions, and adhering to other behavioral regulations. Each of these involves the re-introduction of the integrity of the individual by means of strict control over the person's interaction with the environment.

Upon arrival at the temple and before the worship ceremony (pūjā), the patient must bathe in the pond adjacent to either temple. Since such a requirement is a fairly common one for religious rites, its significance for the curing of pāgalāmi may be minimal. However, that the stereotypic madman is described as one who doesn't bathe perhaps heightens the salient aspect of the ritual bathing. In any event, bathing involves the introduction of a state of ritual purity, signifying the removal of polluting or contaminating external influences. Therefore, bathing is the first step in the re-establishment of the boundaries between individual and environment.

After the curing ceremony, the patient must observe a series of dietary restrictions. Again, dietary prohibitions are a common feature of both ritual activity and of medical treatment procedures. However, as in the case of bathing, it is interesting that the cure entails the reverse process of the disorder: the re-institution of strict regulations to control the introduction of external objects (food) into the individual. Furthermore, the specific injunctions are important. In general, those foods which are prohibited are foods which are "hot" (garama) and which thus stimulate the production of bile (pitta) and heat. This control of "hot" foods is especially clear at Chakrapur where, for the first seven days, the patient is required to eat vegetarian nirāmiṣa food, which is very sāttvika [pure] and which excludes all garama foods. Since pāgalāmi is a disease caused by excess heat, such restrictions make physiological sense within the Ayurvedic framework.

But additionally, "hot" foods are generally rājaṣika, meaning that they are characterized by the guṇa [quality] of rajas [passion].[2] Such foods increase one's passion and activity and consequently, one's attachment to the world. Prohibitions on "hot" foods not only reduce the body heat, but also reduce the passionate energy which attaches the individual to the objects of the material world. "Heat is catalytic in many of these internal processes and external exchanges: it creates an instability that facilitates either separation or combination among particles of different kinds of substances" (Marriott and Inden 1976:12). Conversely, to be "cool" is to be able to withdraw oneself from the external world, to make oneself quiescent and unperturbed by events in the environment. Thus, dietary regulations not only affect the physiological processes responsible for māthāra golamāla, but also aim at restoring the mental state wherein one is immune to environmental intrusiveness of any kind, including "shock," bhara, and tuka. "Coolness" is required not simply to restore humoral equilibrium, but because it has an overall stabilizing effect, enabling the individual to regain the lost distinctive identity.

Besides various food restrictions, temple patients are further restricted from engaging in certain activities. Though the details vary from one temple to the other, nearly all of these injunctions relate to either birth or death. Birth and death are the subject of crucial rites of passage (see Inden and Nicholas, 1977) and thus represent important liminal or transitional phases in the life of an individual (V. Turner, 1967). In addition, they take on even greater significance in the context of the Bengali belief that the individual has a shared bodily relationship with the family:

> The birth or death of one of "one's own people" has been thought of in Bengal as potentially dangerous for both the newborn child or dead person and all those who share his body. This threat to their bodily well-being...comes not from "physical" contact with "polluting" bodily substances, such as blood, afterbirth, or corpses, but from the separation of the bodies involved and the radical transformation which both birth and death are seen to entail. Thus, the periods of impurity are said to start with the separating act which begins the transformation...(Inden and Nicholas 1977: 102-3).

Thus, birth and death are ritual passages not only for the individual who is born or who dies, but for all those persons (i.e., relatives) who share bodily substances with that person. The rituals surrounding these events include a marginal period of liminality during which the relative's own body becomes transformed because of the separation that has occurred. Inden and Nicholas describe this period as akin to death itself:

> During this period, the affected person lacks the competence...to engage in his usual acts of worship; that is, he is unable to come into contact with the gods, and his body is considered untouchable... to others not so affected. One might say that the affected person himself enters a stage approximating death, symbolized by abstinence from certain life-renewing activities such as eating normal food, shaving, changing into fresh clothes, bathing, and the like. The period of impurity ends with the resumption of these activities, all of which may be taken to symbolize his "rebirth" as a normal person (1977:103).

By definition, a rite of passage involves the transformation of the social or moral identity of the individual; within the Bengali context, it also involves the transformation of the material bodily substances which make up the corporal entity of the individual. The liminal period, as that part of the ritual after the termination of one identity and before the assumption of another, is a time when one's identity is ambiguous and "unsettled." As such, it is a period during which the individual is especially "unbounded" and "open" and thus extremely susceptible to disintegrating influences. The temple regulations which direct the patient's behavior at these times emphasize this vulnerability to disintegration. That patient, as one who already suffers from "unboundedness," must be protected from further breakdown.[3]

The most distinctive aspect of the curing ritual at the two temples is the wearing of an iron bangle. Unlike food restrictions and bathing, which are almost inevitable features of ritual activities, the iron bangle is a feature almost unique to this curing ceremony. It is not unreasonable to assume that iron, the strongest and most impenetrable substance known in rural Bengal, is worn in order to strengthen the individual against the very penetration or intrusion which was the cause of the madness ("shock," bhara, or tuka). This interpretation is reinforced by the fact that iron is also used to ward off the possible attack of a bhūta. Just as the power of a mantra can restrain a bhūta from "catching" a victim, the strength of iron can be a similar deterrent.

In this context, it is significant that iron bangles are also required for married women. Women are "softer" than men: "the uterine blood [which predominates in the formation of a female fetus]...is regarded as the source of the 'soft,' unstructured parts of the body: skin, flesh, and blood" (Inden and Nicholas 1977:52). Indeed, the very essence of a married woman is her penetrability, first by her husband and then by her unborn child. Since the key role of a woman is to receive the intrusiveness of her husband and child, it is logical to protect her with an iron bangle from the kind of personal disintegration that happens when one becomes pāgala. Furthermore, it is not merely the woman herself who is thereby protected, but also her husband and her kin group:

> Any fault or normative violation of one person affects not only [her] character, but also those of the other persons with whom [she] shares bodily substances.... [W]hat is affected is not merely the honor or reputation but the very substance of the corporate group and their descendants (Beech 1982:114).

This ethnographic evidence substantiates the view that *pāgalāmi* represents an entropic process, a particular kind of disorder involving the disintegration of the boundaries between the inside and outside which give the individual a unique distinctiveness. Each of the three etiological factors, *bhara*, *tuka*, and "shock," involves an adverse intrusion from the outside environment. Whereas the stereotypic view of the madman emphasizes the loss of those characteristics which serve to regulate interaction with the environment and which thus preserve a sense of individuation and identity, the treatment procedures at the curing temples serve to restore boundaries through restrictions on the patient's interaction with the environment. *Pāgalāmi*, as deviance, signifies a process of entropy due to the loss of the boundaries which differentiate the individual from the environment. *Pāgalāmi* as entropy entails a loss of order and a state of increased chaos, where the regular and ordered relationships among various entities have degenerated.

A Theory of the Person

Both *pāgalāmi* as frustrated desire and *pāgalāmi* as entropy involve the nature of the relationship between the individual and the environment. By environment, I refer to both the "natural world" and the "sociocultural world," and thus to the total configuration of objects, events, and social actors which make up the context within which the individual is situated. I want to explore in more detail the Bengali conception of that relationship between individual and environment and the "theory of the person" which such a relationship implies. *Pāgalāmi* as deviance takes its meaning ultimately from that "theory of the person."

Both the frustrated desire theme and the entropy theme are concerned with the proper relationship between the individual and the environment. In the former, the environment can obstruct the satisfaction of the individual's desires by making the external objects of one's desires unobtainable. Desire, as the classical Sanskritic literature so persuasively argues, is the mode through which the individual becomes attached to the objects of the external world, the motivational impetus for relating to the environment. In this regard, pāgalāmi as deviance signifies the inherent difficulties of that relationship: the gratification of desire depends upon environmental responses which are beyond the control of the individual. The entropy theme underscores another facet of the individual-environment relationship, that the individual's identity is dependent upon boundaries which set apart the individual as a distinctive unit.

Thus, the frustrated desire theme stresses the interdependence of individual and environment, and the entropy theme stresses the need for distinctiveness from the environment. However, while the two themes present differing sides of the individual-environment relationship, both emphasize the individual's existential connection to the surrounding environment. Together, the two conceptions of pāgalāmi underscore the very precariousness of the individual's relationship and the essential paradox of the human situation: establishing relationships while maintaining boundaries.

The frustrated desire theme describes the individual as in constant interaction with the surrounding world. But if the individual is not an isolated, tightly bound unit, is it then reasonable to describe _pāgalāmi_ as entropy in terms of penetration, intrusion, and the loss of distinctiveness through lack of boundary maintenance? The answer is clear if we return to the image of the married woman. Just because she is penetrable, she must be protected against the adverse effects of penetration. Similarly, just because the individual is viewed as an open system in constant interchange with the environment, it is necessary to regulate that interchange. One of the reasons for choosing the term "entropy" is that entropy refers to the relationship between open systems, systems in which there are recurrent transformations of energy and structure. The problem for an open system is to permit interactions and exchanges without the loss of distinctiveness and the consequent dissolution of the system altogether. Thus, just because the individual is not a self-contained entity, _pāgalāmi_ as entropy is a continual possibility. The very open nature of the individual implies _pāgalāmi_ as a form of deviance where the regulation of interchanges has been inadequate, implies _pāgalāmi_ as a process where intrusiveness from the outside erases the differentiation which gives the system its identity.

Together, the two themes of frustrated desire and entropy entail a view of the individual as an open but distinct system within the environment.[4] This representation of the individual is very similar to Marriott and Inden's:

> ...single persons are not ultimately individual units: instead persons are "dividual"; i.e., they are unique composites of diverse subtle and gross substances derived proximately from many and ultimately from one source, and also divisible into separate particles that may be shared or exchanged with others (1976:10).

As an open system, the individual comprises discrete parts, "coded particles...of substances" (Marriott and Inden 1976:10) which form a distinctive structural arrangement and thus give the individual a unique identity. Marriott and Inden refer to this characteristic by saying that persons are "particularized": "they are particular because they are peculiar unique parts of a highly differentiated...order of intersecting natural categories" (1976:10). Marriott and Inden identify such cagories with *jāti*, a Sanskrit word which shares the same etymological roots as the English word "genus" (1976:7). Thus, within Indian thought, the individual has attributes or qualities (*guṇa*) depending upon membership within various cross-cutting genera: geographical, religious, language, sex, occupation, and kinship categories. These *guṇa* make up the unique character of the individual.

As an open system, the individual is continually engaged in interaction with the environment, the view so clearly illustrated through the frustrated desire theme. This interaction is essentially a series of transactions or exchanges between individual and environment involving the "coded particles of substances."

> The coded bodily atoms known to South Asian social thought are acquired by transfers from various sources and are disposed of by transfers toward various destinations. Some substances are acquired originally from the seed and food provided by the parents before birth; others are acquired by later addition through ingestion of food, sexual intercourse, and other means of reception, including sensation. Particles separable from the body (hair, sweat, semen, etc.) are disposed of through excretion and reproduction by the living, and later through the gross and subtle remains of the dead. Persons and genera are thus

> conceived of as channeling and transforming heterogeneous, ever-flowing and changing substances. Living beings naturally and properly seek to acquire better, more appropriate substances for themselves through right eating, right marriages, and other right exchanges and actions (Marriott and Inden 1976:11).

This critical point in the transactional dynamics between individuals and environment must be stressed. Because guṇa (qualities) are always materially embedded, the exchange relationships between individuals and the environment involve those very "atoms" or coded substances which go to make up the identity of the individual. In the language of physics, energy exchanges require structural transformations: the individual's transactions with the environment thus entail the transformation of the individual:

> ...what goes on "between" actors are the same connected processes of mixing and separating that go on "within" actors. Actors' particular natures are thought to be results as well as causes of their particular actions....Varied codes of action or codes of conduct [dharma] are thought to be naturally embodied in actors and otherwise substantiated in the flow of things that pass among actors...Thus, transformations and transactions may be understood as a single set of processes, considered in two ways, internally and externally (Marriott 1976:109-10, 112).

It remains for us to locate pāgalāmi more clearly within this conceptualization of the individual. Pāgalāmi as frustrated desire represents the transactional aspect of the destruction of the individual; pāgalāmi as entropy represents the transformational aspect of the destruction of the individual. They are, therefore, two aspects of the same process. Through passion, the individual is attached to the phenomenal world and is thus at the mercy of environmental forces, "like a boat wafted by the gale" (Bhagavad Gita, quoted in Rao 1962:180). Given this attachment, the frustrated desire theme indicates that pāgalāmi results when transactions with the environment fail to provide an adequate response to the individual's desires. The frustration merely serves to increase the attachment to external objects and to make the individual more vulnerable to the vagaries of environmental responses. Being vulnerable to the environment, the individual becomes less able to maintain the regulations which provide the boundaries enabling separation from the environment. That is, the individual comes to act chaotically within the environment, the extreme being the stereotypic madman who eats anything, lives anywhere, and behaves according to whim.

Transactions with the environment (the frustrated desire theme) imply transformations of the individual (the entropy theme). Since "actions...are thought of as transforming the substances in which they are embodied" (Marriott and Inden 1976:4), action and actor "cannot have separate existences in this world of constituted things" (Marriott 1976:110). To act in the world in a certain way is to become a certain kind of being in the world. As transactions with the environment become random and indiscriminate, the individual's own transformation becomes random and indiscriminate. The individual thus is no longer a distinctive entity. To act indiscriminately and chaotically is to have disrupted those permeable boundaries which separate individual and environment; the result is that one ceases to be a "person" as an entity with a discriminate nature.

This conceptualization helps to make sense of certain religious usages of the word pāgalāmi. For example, a frequent plea included in prayers to Kali is Mā, āmāke pāgala kare dāo ["Mother, make me mad"]. This mystical use of pagalami also involves the concept of the person. A person is one who is attached to the world of external objects and one who has a distinctiveness apart from the environment. Mokṣa or salvation involves liberation and release from just these attributes of the individual -- distinctiveness, and attachment to the world. The plea to Kali is an entreaty to be removed from the binding influence of human desires and to be extinguished as a distinct entity. A clearer translation of the devotee's plea might be "Mother, take away my 'personhood' so that I can be one with You."

Salvation and release provide the solution to the dilemma posed by the individual's interdependent relationship with the environment: freedom from the "clutches" of the external world by extinguishing the passions and desires which bind human beings to the world. However, to accomplish this goal, the individual must also surrender that uniqueness which signifies the status of "person." Indeed, the stereotypic view of the madman might equally well describe the sannyāsī, one who has renounced the world. Like the madman, he eats anything, sleeps anywhere, and does as he pleases.[5] Having attained mokṣa, he need not be concerned with the regulations which guide ordinary people. Earlier, I contrasted mokṣa and pāgalāmi as antithetical categories; but since each involves the annihilation of the person, there is a certain affinity between the two concepts. It is this affinity which enables pāgalāmi to be used as a symbol for mokṣa and, furthermore, which enables both pāgalāmi and mokṣa to represent contrasts to the world of everyday existence.

Pāgalāmi and Madness

I have argued that the theory required to produce pāgalāmi as a social phenomenon is a theory of the person and especially a theory of the relationship between human actors and their environment. It is a theory of the nature of human desire and a theory of the need for boundaries to set the individual apart and make the person a distinctive unit in the world. It is a theory of transactions and of transformations; a theory which views actions as substantiated within actors, and actors as transformed by their actions. It is a theory of the human existential condition; a theory about what it is to be human. This Bengali theory can be compared with the conception of madness in the West.

The Western conception of madness reflects the strict dualistic dichotomy maintained between nature and culture.[6] The mad person is not merely a-cultural, but is also naturalized. Within an ideology which came increasingly to identify human beings as rational, madness is seen as being devoid of reason. Having lost that which makes one distinctively human, the mad person is reduced to the animal level. Madness, as deviance, is a potent indication of an individual's loss of reason, of mind, of culture: and ultimately, of the loss of humanity itself.

But madness does not, in the Western conception, simply happen to people. Fundamentally, it is something that is within all individuals. There is a deep fear of madness, not as something "out there," but as something within the individual which remains a perpetual possibility. To prevent its actualization, madness must be kept under control. In a very meaningful sense, madness is a form of letting go and of going out of control. It is this conception of madness as an ever-present potential requiring careful surveillance which leads to the Western obsession with confining madness, in the concrete form of the mad person, within the physical constraints of the asylum.

If madness represents the loss of reason and a de-culturation of human beings, then it is easy to understand this fear of madness as a potentiality within the individual. For, however much reason or mind makes human beings distinctive, humans also incorporate nature. It is this animal nature which, when uncontrolled by reason, is expressed in madness, as exemplified in the Western stereotypic image of the violent aggression and sexuality of the mad person. Having lost one's reason, the mad person has lost the cultural means for controlling and subduing that basic animal nature.

Madness arises out of the struggle between human culture and human "nature." The two are in conflict, and madness warns of the consequences when the latter overthrows the former. The Western ideology dichotomizes nature and culture but then inserts them both within human beings. Human personality becomes the battleground for the dominance of one principle over another, and the distinctiveness of human beings from the animal world is only maintained if culture dominates. Thus, the mad person not only represents the failure of humanity and the consequent reduction to the animal level, but also is an indication of that very possibility happening to all. Because madness is a basic human potentiality, it is never far away, however carefully it might be confined.

The distinctive attributes of madness -- as potentiality within the individual, as uncontrolled aggression and sexuality, and as an intense internal conflict -- are rooted in the basic dualities of Western thought: nature/culture, mind/body, reason/passion. That pāgalāmi fails to exhibit such qualities is further indication that these dualities are not part of the Bengali experience. Whereas madness rests on a conceptualization of human beings as incorporating two antithetical principles, pāgalāmi derives from a conceptualization of the individual as an open system in interaction with the surrounding environment. Madness is a potentiality within the individual, but pāgalāmi is a potentiality which threatens to obliterate the individual.

Yet, in spite of these contrasts, both concepts inform us of the basic human existential situation as conceived by each culture. Both madness and pāgalāmi are implicated in the respective conceptions of human beings, and represent deviance in a very ultimate sense. The mad person, through the loss of reason, descends into the animal realm; the pāgala, through entropy, is reduced to the primeval homogeneity. But both are de-humanized and both lose their distinctive identities as human beings.

Because both madness and pāgalāmi illustrate human deviance in this ultimate sense, they also provide answers to fundamental questions regarding human nature and the individual's relationship to the outside world. How are human beings part of the world and yet unique? How are they part of nature and yet distinctive? The Western answer builds on a dichotomy between nature and culture, with human participation in both realms providing both unity with and uniqueness from the surrounding world. Without this basic duality, the Bengali view envisions human beings as part of the all-encompassing natural-moral order. Differentiation is, then, effected through open boundaries and the controlled regulation of interchanges between various units of the total system. If the Western conceptual problem is to build bridges between two mutually exclusive and incompatible categories, then the Bengali problem is to erect fences within an all-inclusive and primordial homogeneity. In both cases, madness and *pāgalāmi* demonstrate how tenuous bridges and fences can be.

NOTES

1. The Bengali word *pāgala* [mad person] does not indicate gender. The stereotype I describe seems to apply to both men and women. However, in my experience, almost all of those who do live on the streets are men, and therefore I have used the masculine English word.

2. Some informants cite two exceptions; *ghi* [clarified butter] and *ātapa-cala* [a particular type of rice] are both *garama* [hot] and *sāttvika* [pure]. They can cause *peta garama* ["hot stomach," stomachache] but not a *garama mejāja* [hot temperament].

3. Significantly, *rājasika* food is prohibited during the mourning period. This point reinforces the earlier one that avoidance of *rājasika* food helps to stabilize the individual. The widow seems to be considered especially vulnerable and must abstain from *rājasika* food for the rest of her life.

The general prohibition for Chakrapur patients on eating at a *karma bārī* [ceremonial house] is also relevant in this context. A *karma bārī* is a house where one of the various *samskāra* [rites of passage] is taking place. As Inden and Nicholas (1977:66) point out, "Any act that changes the status of a person by transforming his body (and his inherent code of conduct) may be classified by Bengalis as an act of birth. All *samskāra* meet this qualification."

4. There is evidence that units other than the individual are conceived as open systems and thus require regulations regarding their transactions with the surrounding environment. In his study of the nature of transactions within Hindu society, Marriott (1976) notes the different transactions which characterize different caste groups and different religious cults as well as the four stages of life. Similarly, Inden and Nicholas's (1977) exploration of Bengali kinship stresses the nature of kin groups as open systems. The discussions of birth and death are illustrative of the kin group as an open system. But undoubtedly the most dramatic example of this concern with boundary maintenance is the marriage ritual, wherein a woman must be transformed into the same bodily substance as her husband before she can be incorporated into the new kin unit. As such, it is also the second birth for a woman. A third example is Beech's (1982)

analysis of the "domestic realm" and the Bengali home. The physical and structural openness of the house with respect to the environment contrasts sharply with the ritual segregation that demonstrates the importance of house boundaries. _Pāgalāmi_ specifically refers to the collapse of the boundaries between the inside and outside of the individual, but it could be hypothesized that other categories of deviance would denote boundary violations and entropic processes within other system-units of Bengali society.

5. Illustrative is the story of a sage who lived in Benares during the time of British rule. After he was invited to dinner at the home of an important British officer, he reciprocated the invitation. When the officer was shocked to find that the meal consisted of human feces, the sage replied, "But Sahib, food or shit, it is all the same to me." This extreme non-discrimination characterizes both madman and holy man.

6. Though this analysis draws on Foucault (1965), it relies on my own reflection on what madness is. Therefore, this comparison must remain tentative until Western conceptions have been researched more thoroughly.

APPENDICES

APPENDIX A

Star Descriptions

1. I'm thinking of a man -- let's call him Frank Jones -- who is very suspicious; he doesn't trust anybody, and he's sure that everybody is against him. Sometimes he thinks that people he sees on the street are talking about him or following him around. A couple of times now, he has beaten up men who didn't even know him. The other night, he began to curse his wife terribly; then he hit her and threatened to kill her because, he said, she was working against him too, just like everybody else.

2. Now here's a young woman in her twenties, let's call her Betty Smith...she has never had a job, and she doesn't seem to want to go out and look for one. She is a very quiet girl; she doesn't talk much to anyone -- even her own family, and she acts like she is afraid of people, especially young men her own age. She won't go out with anyone, and whenever someone comes to visit her family, she stays in her own room until they leave. She just stays by herself and daydreams all the time, and shows no interest in anything or anybody.

3. Here's another kind of man; we can call him George Brown. He has a good job and is doing pretty well at it. Most of the time he gets along all right with people, but he is always very touchy and he always loses his temper quickly, if things aren't going his way, or if people find fault with him. He worries a lot about little things, and he seems to be moody and unhappy all the time. Everything is going along all right for him, but he can't sleep nights, brooding about the past, and worrying about things that might go wrong.

4. How about Bill Williams? He never seems to be able to hold a job very long, because he drinks so much. Whenever he has money in his pocket, he goes on a spree; he stays out till all hours drinking, and never seems to care what happens to his wife and children. Sometimes he feels very bad about the way he treats his family; he begs his wife to forgive him and promises to stop drinking, but he always goes off again.

5. Here's a different sort of girl -- let's call her Mary White. She seems happy and cheerful; she's pretty, has a good job, and is engaged to marry a nice young man. She has loads of friends; everybody likes her, and she's

always busy and active. However, she just can't leave the house without going back to see whether she left the gas stove lit or not. And she always goes back again, just to make sure she locked the door. And one other thing about her: she's afraid to ride up and down in elevators; she just won't go anyplace where she'd have to ride in an elevator to get there.

6. Now, I'd like to describe a 12-year-old boy -- Bobby Grey. He's bright enough and in good health, and he comes from a comfortable home. But his father and mother have found out that he's been telling lies for a long time now. He's been stealing things from stores, and taking money from his mother's purse, and he has been playing truant, staying away from school whenever he can. His parents are very upset about the way he acts, but he pays no attention to them.

(from Dohrenwend and Chin-Shong 1967:418-19)

APPENDIX B

Interviewing Clients

A fundamental paradox within the sociology of knowledge is that studying knowledge involves formulating knowledge about knowledge. Thus, knowledge is both the topic of the research (Bengali knowledge) and the product of the research (my knowledge about Bengali knowledge). To be consistent, I must apply the same theoretical approach to my own knowledge that I have adopted to examine Bengali ethnopsychiatric knowledge: knowledge is the result of social processes and must be described within the context of those social activities. Thus, the researcher has a constructivistic role both in creating the data and in developing the analysis. Data are constituted through the process by which the researcher selects certain observable phenomena as relevant, dismisses other observations as irrelevant, and analytically links one phenomenon with another.

If this constructivist role of the researcher is acknowledged -- and my orientation to the sociology of knowledge dictates that it must be -- then it is essential to discuss methodology as an integral part of the findings. As a researcher who is producing knowledge, I must acknowledge my own actions and interests and how these construct the research findings. Knowledge cannot be separated from the knowing of it. As I examine the following interview, the concern is an analysis of my knowing in order to contextualize the discussion of my research findings.[1]

The interview is one that my assistant and I conducted with relatives of an outpatient at the Bhowanipore Mental Observation Ward, a well-known allopathic clinic in Calcutta. Because of its spacious and attractive gardens, Bhowanipore does not seem to be in the middle of congested Calcutta. The inner and outer courtyards are separated by a row of offices, including the outpatient examination rooms. My interviews took place in a room at the very end of the open corridor connecting the offices. The client, an elderly peasant, had brought his son from their village home outside Calcutta.

> I cultivate my own land. I can read a little Bengali -- such as the newspaper. My son passed Class X. After that, his head became like this.

[When did that happen?]

It began about six months ago. Since three years ago, a lot has happened. Occasionally, it happens and then he becomes well. A folk healer was seen; he gave some medicine, but nothing happened. One day, he had gone far away to catch fish and returned at night. In the morning, he suddenly laughed a lot. He said, 'I saw this; I saw that.' He spoke nonsense, began to hit, and didn't want to eat. He had to be forced to eat. When well, he says nothing.

[Was any medicine given or did he become better on his own?]

He became better on his own. I gave him green coconut water to drink because his body was hot, but nothing happened.

[Is he always like this or only sometimes?]

It increases in winter.

[Why did you bring him here?]

There is a doctor there where I live. Getting the information from him, I came here.

[How does he behave at home?]

At home he creates disturbances. He fears me and he loves me. Some people say that it is 'evil glance'; some say it is a head malfunctioning. I don't know what it is.

[My assistant turns to me to see if there are any more questions, and then begins to thank the respondent and to dismiss him. The client interrupts.]

> He does not sleep well. He does not move his bowels. His urine is red. And he doesn't urinate much. When it increases, then it becomes like this. He is given water from soaking chick peas, water from soaking the bark of the nima tree, and green coconut water.

An analysis of this interview must begin with Schutz's concept of "systems of relevances." In his discussion of everyday knowledge, Schutz argues that an individual's system of relevances establishes a selective attention to the world. Relevances are established by the actor's interest or "purpose-at-hand"; it is "interest that breaks asunder the unproblematic field of the preknown into various zones of various relevance with respect to such interest" (1970:111-12). My own interests with regard to analyzing the interviews are clear: to generate knowledge in relation to the conception of mental illness in Bengal. This interest is so broad, however, that it is difficult to connect it to the construction of data and the consequent research findings.

One of the reasons for choosing this particular interview is that my purpose-at-hand can be defined more narrowly and concretely, thus making it easier to perceive the link between that interest and the research conclusions. At the time of the interview, I wondered why the man interrupted the "dismissal" to provide additional information [lines 33-40]. Thus, my purpose-at-hand in the analysis was to answer why the respondent made a particular point of giving us the additional information. Since it is that question which prompted me to analyze the interview, I want to first discuss how that interest or purpose-at-hand was established so that the question was formulated as a problematic issue requiring analysis.

Since the medical purposes of the allopathic psychiatric clinic are clearly communicated to the clients, it can be assumed that this man identified my purposes as those of the clinic, namely, to give medical care to his son. Therefore, he probably perceived me as occupying the role of specialist in a psychiatric interactional sequence. As a specialist, I was accorded a superordinate position and the authority to determine the topic of conversation and what was relevant to that conversation. The interactional norms of the situation specified that I was to ask questions and the client was to answer. Consequently, this particular man violated those norms by interrupting our dismissal and continuing the interview. My research assistant and I commented on this unusual behavior as a breach of our expectations.[2]

Yet, while I noticed the violation, I also felt that the father himself did not view his behavior as a breach. His previously respectful and polite demeanor made me hesitant to conclude that he was refusing to accept our authority to direct the interview. Therefore, I understood his remarks to mean "this is something relevant and important to your purposes, and thus to the medical treatment of my son." When he described a series of fairly common symptoms and folk remedies, my reaction was that the information was not really important. I was therefore faced with conflicting data: hearing the father say "this is important," and observing him giving inconsequential information. This discrepancy constituted my inability to make sense of what was being said, thus raising a problematic issue requiring further analysis.

When I examined the informational content more closely, I learned that all three of the home remedies he mentioned are believed to have a cooling effect. This observation and the father's mention of the son's body being hot illustrate the "burning sensation" syndrome that Chakraborty (1971) noted among Bengali psychiatric patients. According to Ayurveda, pitta or bile contains the heat of the body, and thus its disruption produces a burning sensation. Furthermore, other statements can be interpreted within the Ayurvedic humoral perspective. "Red urine," referring to very concentrated, strong urine, is also a symptom of humoral imbalance. In addition, the father's comment that the boy's symptoms increased in winter is relevant to Ayurvedic belief that there are particular seasons and times of day when each of the humors is likely to become deranged. Thus, the father described his son's illness within a contemporary popular version of Ayurveda in which the hot-cold dimension is an important symptom in diagnosing disease. The medical events he noticed are those which are relevant to Ayurvedic theory. In constituting his son as being ill, the father was attending to those features of the situation which might be legitimate within Ayurvedic medicine.[3] Therefore, we can conclude that the additional information he gave owed its significance to the Ayurvedic interpretation of disease he was using.

However, this conclusion does not explain the client's urgency to provide the needed information, i.e., his refusal to be dismissed before presenting it. At the time of the interview, I was struck by the juxtaposition of māthāra golamāla [malfunctioning of the head] and apaḍr̥ṣṭi [literally, inauspicious glance; referring to possession]: "some people say that it is apadṛṣṭi; some say it is māthāra golamāla. I don't know what it is." The father is acknowledging two alternative characterizations of the boy's condition: the case might be an instance of apadṛṣṭi or of māthāra golamāla. Such a disagreement about diagnosis assumes that the two are mutually exclusive alternatives; therefore, one cannot be the cause of the other. This conclusion was significant for me, because at the time of the interview, I thought that māthāra golamāla was a general term for madness and apadṛṣṭi one of several causal agents of madness.

I was also puzzled by the father's statement that his son went fishing and returned late the night before falling ill. At this point in the analysis, it remained inexplicable. But again, before asking why the father included this information, it is necessary to examine how this question itself emerged and therefore to reexamine the social context of the interview. A father has brought his son to an allopathic clinic to receive treatment as a mental patient. Thus, in order to achieve his purpose-at-hand, he must somehow establish a sense that this is an instance of mental illness. Only in this way can the father account for and justify his appeal for treatment.[4] The father's task, therefore, is to select and organize a series of verbal statements so that in their entirety, they accomplish this purpose. Of all the possible things which he could conceivably relate about his son, he must select those very items which enable him to accomplish the statement, "This person is mentally ill and requires treatment."

Our task as analysts is just the reverse. Our task is to inspect the outcome, the respondent's talk, in term of how such an account has been produced, in terms of how he has methodically organized his speech utterances. From this perspective, it becomes pertinent to ask why the respondent provides us with this particular information. We must ask how his statements, individually and as a whole, enable him to produce an instance of mental illness. Since the father's speech is a methodical production stemming from his purpose-at-hand (i.e., his need to justify his appeal for treatment by demonstrating that his son is mentally ill), we must conclude that the father told us about the fishing incident because he thinks it is relevant to his son's illness.

As I puzzled over the possible significance of the fishing story, a fortuitous event occurred. I had been using the Ayurvedic paradigm for understanding the interview and had almost given up hope that I could make sense of the comment about going fishing. As I discussed my research with a Bengali friend, he said, "But don't you see? That's when he became possessed by the ghost!" He then explained that not only is one category of ghosts specifically called mechō bhūta [fish ghosts], but that ghosts of all kinds are very fond of fish. In fact, to say, "those who like fish" is a sufficient reference to identify ghosts, and often a necessary circumlocution when pronouncing their names at night might attract the ghosts. Ghosts are also known to be especially active at night in seeking out their victims. It is now obvious why the father suspects possession: the young man went fishing and returned late at night, two things which suggest the possibility of attracting the attention of ghosts.

Other aspects of the interview are comprehensible within the context of suspected ghost possession. The father consulted an ōjhā to exorcise the ghost. The patient's statement, "I have seen this one; I have seen that one" probably refers to the angry ghosts attacking him. Finally, the father indicates that his son's personality has changed: "At home he creates disturbances. He fears me and he loves me." Since the ghost has taken over the victim's body, the possessed person has become the vehicle for the ghost's personality. Aggression, talking nonsense, and sleeplessness are all signs of the ghost's presence.

To conclude the analysis of this interview, an examination of the internal structure of the interview helps to integrate the preceding observations. The interview can be divided into four parts. The first five lines include responses to our initial introductory questions, which were designed to elicit basic socioeconomic data. The next section (lines 6-18), in response to the question "When did that happen?" is the ghost story. After directly answering our question, the respondent proceeds to tell us what he did, why he did it, and what the results were. The third part begins where the father is asked if medicine was given, and continues until the accepted dismissal (lines 19-32). The final section (lines 33-40) is the added information we are trying to explain, organized around the Ayurvedic conceptualization. In summary, the interview consists of introduction, ghost account, question-answer repartee, and Ayurvedic theme. Our original question can then be reformulated as, "Why was the fourth section, the Ayurvedic theme, so crucial that the respondent refused to accept our dismissal until he had included it?"

As noted, the father's task during the interview is to present his son as an instance of mental illness in order to account for this request for treatment at the allopathic clinic. Unless he can do so, his request will be meaningless and his efforts will have been wasted. We can therefore conclude that the father did not see his interruption of our dismissal as a social violation because the Ayurvedic theme was essential for justifying his appeal for treatment. This conclusion reinforces the previous distinction between apadṛṣṭi and māthāra golamāla. Though a construction of an instance of possession does produce "my son is mad," it does not justify the son's treatment at the clinic, for possession requires a different form of treatment, an ōjhā's exorcism of the ghost. Such a procedure, the father told us, had failed to have any effect. Confronted with the ineffectiveness of that treatment, the alternative of head malfunctioning became more probable and the father thus sought treatment for such a possibility. But at the time of our attempted dismissal, the father had been unable to prsent his son as an instance of māthāra golamāla, and so he had to continue the interview with the Ayurvedic theme, giving the symptoms which suggest māthāra golamāla. Only now has he produced a description of his son as one requiring the medical treatment available at the allopathic clinic.

Finally, I want to explicitly acknowledge some of the methodological assumptions and procedures used in this analysis. Of primary significance is the assumption that the respondent's talk is purposeful and that understanding that talk requires recognizing the purposes at-hand and relevances of the speaker. That is, since the respondent is trying to do something by means of his speech utterance (R. Turner, 1974; Labov and Fanshel, 1977), the identification of that "doing" is important for a full comprehension of what is said. This assumption implies the necessity to focus on the speech or communication activity itself rather than merely on the abstract cognitive content of the words and sentences. That content is introduced within the total social context and thus must be analyzed as a situated production within that context.[5]

This particular point, the methodological importance and use of a respondent's interests and relevances, is simply an instance of the more general principle that research activity is one kind of social praxis. In order to understand such situated social interaction, the analyst must explicitly acknowledge the social setting and the interactional constraints it entails, as well as the actors and their pre-interactional frames of reference. Thus, for example, the researcher plays a far from passive role in the research process. In order to "hear" the respondent at all, the researcher must make assumptions about what the interaction will be like (e.g., he/she must assume that they are talking about madness). These assumptions influence the researcher's speech activity, are communicated to the respondent, and thus influence the whole interaction process. Similarly, within the analysis, the researcher approaches the data with certain interests and relevances which affect what the researcher attends to and "sees" in the data. Because knowledge is embedded in the social praxis which generates it, the research product must be located within the particular social praxis, the research process, from which it was derived. The social factors of the situation, actors, interaction, and analytic activity must be examined explicitly within the methodological procedures used to reach research conclusions and to thereby construct knowledge. The analysis of this sample interview has demonstrated how this goal can be achieved in a fairly explicit and rigorous manner.

NOTES

1. The best example of this analytic technique is Labov and Fanshel's (1977) analysis of therapeutic discourse. While I was not familiar with their work when I first did my analysis in the field, they note that they had been influenced by the work of Harvey Sacks, whose work I have also used (1972, 1974). See also Zimmerman, 1974.

2. However, during other interviews, instances of such violations often went unnoticed. These breaches differed from the present one in that they entailed some additional statement which explained or excused the breach. For example, a client might say, "do you want to know about..." or, "maybe it is important that...." The breach is thereby introduced by a device which acknowledges it and accounted for it in terms of the possible significance of the information to be supplied. In contrast, this father simply interrupted my assistant. Because he did not attempt to normalize his interruption to keep it within the confines of the interactional norms of the interview, it was a noticeable violation of those norms.

This interview, therefore, contrasts rather sharply with another incident. The psychiatrist inadvertently sent a relative whom we had interviewed several weeks earlier. We explained that since we had already talked with her, it was unnecessary for us to do so again. She replied, "that day, I forgot to tell you something," thereby constituting her possible breach as legitimate and also aligning herself with our purposes (the obtaining of information about the patient).

3. This concept of "legitimate symptoms" is applicable to any medical system. A personal anecdote comes to mind. When my daughter fell ill in India, with a general complaint of stomach pain and an enlarged spleen, I finally took her to a specialist. Beforehand, I composed a "case history," carefully trying to include everything of medical significance of the past month. At the consultation, the doctor asked me if she had had any skin rashes. I replied, "no," but my daughter reminded me that she had had a rash on her neck. My comment was, "Oh, that was just a bit of heat rash." Since I had, in my own mind, already accounted for the rash, it was not a legitimate symptom of the present complaint and I no longer "attended" to it.

4. If his son had been present, the father could have used his son's immediate behavior in our presence for such a construction of an instance of mental illness. That is, the father could have indicated the son's illness by simply pointing to the presumed symptom: "he does THAT." Such a technique is particularly interesting because it assumes that the other (the psychiatrist, a relative, myself) in the interaction understands what "that" is and thus shares an intersubjective frame of reference. For exactly this reason, i.e., that I could not assume that the respondent and I shared the same frame of reference, I always asked the patient to wait outside. This strategy forces the respondent to verbalize his descriptions, giving me more information about his own definition of the situation.

5. Although I have focused on a single purpose-at-hand in this interview, it is clearly purposeful in multiple ways. For example, the father's talk also serves to structure the authority relationship between us. In fact, this purpose -- the respondent's concern about structuring the relationship between the respondent and myself -- often interfered with the research task. Direct questions such as "How do people become mad?" often fail to elicit relevant responses because the respondent's talk is organized by the need to structure our relationship (e.g., to demonstrate hospitality or to assert a superordinate position). Thus a good methodological principle is to structure situations in which the relevances of the researcher coincide with the respondent's (suspected) purpose-at-hand.

APPENDIX C

Glossary of Bengali and Sanskrit Terms

abhāva. Insufficiency, need

āghāta. Blow, either physical or mental

ambala. A sour drink

annaprāśana. "First rice" ceremony for infants

apadṛṣṭi. Literally, inauspicious glance; ghost possession

apaghāta-mṛityu. "Unnatural death"; death "before one's time" or by accident

apasmāra. Epilepsy

ārogya bālā. Curing bangle; the bangle given at the temple after the patient is cured

artha. Wealth, economic prosperity; one of the four ultimate aims of mortal life

aśānti. Disharmony, unhappiness

āśrama. Stage of life; the four *āśrama* are *brahmacārī* [apprentice], *gṛhastha* [householder], *vānaprastha* [hermit], and *sannyāsī* [ascetic mendicant]

asukha. Disease, illness

asustha. Unwell, sick, ill

asvābhāvika. Unnatural, abnormal

ātapa-cala. A particular kind of rice

ā̃ṭura-ghara. Birth-room; the room reserved for the delivery of a baby

bak-bak. Nonsense, gibberish

bālā. Heavy bangle

bāṇamārā. Literally, striking with an arrow; a technique for tuka [sorcery], where a dream figure is pierced with an arrow to cause his or her death

bāṛī. House, home

bāṛīra bau. Wife of the house; a woman married to one of the men in the household

bhara. Possession by a spirit, ghost, etc

bhūta. Ghost, dead person who cannot leave the earthly world

bhūta bhara. Ghost possession

bhūte pāoyā. Ghost possession

bhūtonmāda. Ghost madness; insanity caused by a ghost

boāla. A variety oflarge fish

bojhā. Reason, understanding

brahmacārī. Apprentice, student; the first of the āśrama, stages of life

buddhi. Intellect, judgment

cikitsā. Treatment, therapy

cintā. Thought, worry, anxiety

ḍāktāra. Doctor; can refer to allopathic, homeopathic, or Ayurvedic practitioners

deśa. Country

dharma. Duty, moral code, the law; one of the four ultimate aims of mortal life

dhātu. Bodily component: food juice, blood, flesh, fat, bone, marrow, and semen

doṣa.	Humor of the body: vāyu [wind], pitta [bile], kapha [phlegm]
duḥkha.	Sorrow
dūṣita hāōyā.	Polluted or poisoned breeze, thought to cause madness
garama.	Hot (in temperature)
garama mejāja.	Literally, hot temperament; a volatile temperament, easy to anger
ghāṭa.	Riverside landing; the burning ghāṭa is the place along the river where the funeral pyres are erected
ghi.	Clarified butter
gṛhastha.	Householder; the second of the āśrama or stages of life
guṇa.	Quality, attribute
guṇina.	A person with special qualities or skills; another name for ōjhā [folk healer]
guru.	Teacher
hākima.	Practitioner of Unani medicine
jāgrata.	Awake, lively; used to refer to a potent and responsive form of a deity, especially Kali
jala paṛā.	To sprinkle the patient with water into which special power has been infused by reciting mantra [verses]
jāti.	Genus, caste

jhāṛa phuk. Magical ritual involving blowing on the patient while reciting mantra [verses]

jñāti. Blood relatives

kāla. Time, historical period

kāma. Passion, erotic desire; one of the four ultimate aims of mortal life

kapha. Phlegm; one of the three doṣa [bodily humors]

karma bāṛī. Ceremonial house; a house where one of the saṃskāra [rites of passage] is taking place

kavaca. Amulet, talisman

kavirāja. An Ayurvedic practitioner

khāoyā. Eating; food consumption

kheyāla khuśī. Inclination, whim

māduli. Amulet, talisman

mana. Mind; seat of understanding. Also, manas

mana khārāpa. Literally, bad mind; depression, sadness

mānasika. Vow, religious promise

mānasika dvanda. Mental conflict

manera āghāta. Literally, blow to the mind; a mental blow or upset

mantra. Words or syllables often without overt meaning, believed to have a magico-sacred power

mantragupti. "Hidden" or secret mantra, verses

mantrapūta. Blessed with mantra

mantraśakti. The power of a mantra

māthā-garama. Literally, hot head; mad, crazy

māthā-khārāpa. Literally, bad head; mad, crazy

māthāradoṣa. Literally, defect of the head; madness, mental illness

māthāra golamāla. Literally, malfunctioning or disturbance of the head; mental illness

māyā. Illusion

mechō-bhūta. A ghost which loves fish and stays near bodies of water

melā. Fair, carnival

mokṣa. Release, liberation, salvation; one of the four ultimate aims of mortal life

murcchā. Epilepsy

nawab. Muslim ruler of a province

nima. A variety of margosa tree; a common habitat for *bhūta* [ghosts]; the water from soaking the bark is believed to be very cooling

nirāmiṣa. "Pure" food; excludes meat, fish, eggs, garlic, onions, and one variety of lentils

ōjhā. Folk healer, exorcist

oṣudha. Medicine; can also refer to the potion given by a sorcerer

pāgala. (adj.) Mad, crazy, mentally ill; (noun) a mad person (pl., *pāgalarā*)

pāgalāmi. Madness, insanity, mental illness

peṭa garama.	"Hot" stomach, stomachache
pitta.	Bile; one of the three *doṣa* or bodily humors
pretātmā.	The self of a dead person
pūjā.	Prayer ritual; religious worship
pũṭi.	A variety of small fish
rajas.	Energy, passion; one of the three *guṇa* [qualities] (adj., *rājaṣika*)
rasa.	Taste
rogī.	Patient. Also, *rugi*
rojā.	Variant of *ōjhā* [folk healer]
sādha.	Intense desire or craving; the ritual during pregnancy where the woman's desires are to be fulfilled
sādhu.	Holy man
śāka.	Green leafy vegetable, such as spinach or mustard greens
śakti.	Power, strength (both physical and mental)
saṃskāra.	Rite of passage; in contemporary Bengal, includes *sādha* [pre-birth ritual]; *annaprāśana* [first-rice ceremony for infants]; *paitā* [sacred thread ceremony]; *biye* [marriage]; and *śrāddha* [funeral]
sannyāsī.	An ascetic mendicant; the *āśrama* or stage of life when ties to the world are renounced
sārā.	Cure, curing

sattva. Existence, purity; one of the three *guṇa* or qualities. (adj., *sāttvika*)

śiṅgi. A variety of freshwater fish

śoka. Intense grief, such as at the death of a loved one

śola. A variety of large fish

śrāddha. Funeral ceremony

srota. Pathways, channels

svadharma. Personal duty; one's own moral code

tamas. Inertia, ignorance; one of the three *guṇa* [qualities]. (adj., *tāmasika*)

ṭhāṇḍā. Cool, cold (in temperature)

ṭhāṇḍā mejāja. Literally, cool temperament; even, calm temperament

ṭola. Traditional Sanskrit school; school for Ayurvedic practitioners

tridoṣa. Three humors of the body: *vāyu* [wind], *pitta* [bile], and *kapha* [phlegm]

tuka. Sorcery, evil spell

tukatāka. Another word for *tuka* [sorcery]

ucche. The vegetable bitter squash

unmāda. (noun) insanity, mania; (adj.) insane, manic, crazy

utarāna. To pass a test successfully, hence, to complete the training for becoming an *ōjhā* [folk healer]

vānaprastha.	Hermit; the third āśrama or stage of life
varṇa.	One of the principal social classes described in early Sanskrit literature, e.g., Brahmana, Ksatriya
vāyu.	Wind; one of the three doṣa [bodily humors]. Also, vāta

BIBLIOGRAPHY

Austin, J.L.
1962 How to Do Things with Words. Cambridge: Harvard University Press.

Bagadia, V.N. et al.
1973 Depression: family and psychodynamic study of 233 cases. Indian Journal of Psychiatry 15:217-23.

Bang, B.G.
1973 Current concepts of the smallpox goddess Sitala in parts of West Bengal. Man in India 53(1):79-97.

Basham, A.L.
1959 The Wonder That Was India: A Survey of the Culture of the Indian Sub-Continent Before the Coming of the Muslims. New York: Grove Press.

1976 The practice of medicine in ancient and medieval India. In Asian Medical Systems: A Comparative Study. Charles Leslie, ed. Pp. 18-43. Berkeley: University of California Press.

Beals, A.L.
1976 Strategies of resort to curers in South India. In Asian Medical Systems: A Comparative Study. Charles Leslie, ed. Pp. 184-200. Berkeley: University of California Press.

Becker, Howard S.
1963 Outsiders: Studies in the Sociology of Deviance. New York: The Free Press.

Beech, Mary Higdon
1976 "The cultural definition of a Bengali meal." Paper presented at the Twelth Annual Bengal Studies Conference, University of Michigan, Ann Arbor.

1982 The domestic realm in the lives of Hindu women in Calcutta. In Separate Worlds: Studies of Purdah in South Asia. Hanna Papanek and Gail Minault, eds. Pp. 110-38. Delhi: Chanakya Publications.

Berger, Peter L. and Thomas Luckmann
1966 The Social Construction of Reality: A Treatise in the Sociology of Knowledge. Garden City, NY: Doubleday.

Berreman, Gerald D.
1964 Brahmins and shamans in Pahari religion. In Religion in South Asia. Edward B. Harper, ed. Pp. 53-70. Seattle: University of Washington Press.

Bhardwaj, S.M.
1973 Early phase of homeopathy in India. Asian Profile 1:281-96.

Bhowmick, P.K.
1973 Functioning secret institutions. Proceedings of the Sixtieth Indian Science Congress, Chandigarh: Section on Anthropology and Archaeology, Presidental Address.

Bittner, Egon
1973 Objectivity and realism in sociology. In Phenomenological Sociology: Issues and Applications. George Psathas, ed. Pp. 109-28. New York: John Wiley and Sons.

Blum, Alan F.
1970 The sociology of mental illness. In Deviance and Respectability: The Social Construction of Moral Meanings. Jack D. Douglas, ed. Pp. 31-60. New York: Basic Books.

Bose, Grinindrasekher
1945 Everyday Psychoanalysis. Calcutta: Susil Gupta.

1966 A New Theory of Mental Life. Calcutta: Indian Psychoanalytic Association.

Brar, H.S.
1970 Yoga and psychoanalysis. British Journal of Psychiatry 116:201-6.

Carstairs, G. Morris
1955 Medicine and faith in rural Rajasthan. In Health, Culture, and Community: Case Studies of Public Reactions to Health Programs. Benjamin D. Paul, ed. Pp. 107-34. New York: Russell Sage Foundation.

1956 Hinjra and jiryan: two derivatives of Hindu attitudes to sexuality. British Journal of Medical Psychology 29:128-38.

Carstairs, G. Morris
1957 The Twice Born: A Study of a Community of High Caste Hindus. London: The Hogarth Press.

Chakrabarti, Prafulla
1973 Some observations on the pilgrims and their pilgrimages: Tarakeswar. Human Events 7(7):17-29.

Chakraborty, Ajita
1970 Directory of Mental Health Activities in India. Calcutta: Indian Psychiatric Society.

Chakraborty, Ajita
1971 Origin of a common psychiatric symptom (burning sensations) among Indian patients: study of a myth with reference to Ayurveda. Paper presented at the Fifth World Congress of Psychiatry, Mexico City.

Chakraborty, Ajita and Amal Mallick
1966 Headache (a cross-cultural study). Indian Journal of Psychiatry 8:101-8.

Chatterjee, Acharya Prabhakar
1972 My experiments with cuckoo's meat in the treatment of mental diseases. Journal of Research in Indian Medicine 7(2):79-81.

Clements, Forrest E.
1932 Primitive concepts of disease. University of California Publications in American Archaeology and Ethnology 32:185-252.

Coster, Geraldine
1934 Yoga and Western Psychotherapy: A Comparison. London: Oxford University Press.

Davis, Marvin
1976a The individual among Bengali Hindus. Man in India 56:189-214.

1976b A philosophy of Hindu rank from rural West Bengal. Journal of Asian Studies 36:5-24.

De Bary, William Theodore, ed.
1958 Sources of Indian Tradition, Vol. 1. New York: Columbia University Press.

Deshmukh, D.R.
1972 Experiments in the management of psychological disorders with yoga. Journal of the Yoga Institute 18(5):80-83.

Dimock, Edward C., Jr. and Ronald Inden
1969 Problems of Transliteration in Bengal Studies. In Bengal East and West. A. Lipski, ed. Pp. 11-17. East Lansing: Michigan State University, Asian Studies Center, South Asia Series Occasional Paper No. 13.

Dohrenwend, Bruce P. and Edwin Chin-Shong
1967 Social status and attitudes toward psychological disorder: the problem of tolerance of deviance. American Sociological Review 32:417-33.

Epstein, Scarlett
1974 Social analysis of witch beliefs in a Mysore village. In Tribe, Caste, and Peasantry. K.S. Mathur and B.C. Agarwal, eds. Pp. 361-74. Lucknow: The Ethnographic and Folk Culture Society, U.P.

Erikson, Kai T.
1966 Wayward Puritans: A Study in the Sociology of Deviance. New York: John Wiley and Sons.

Evans-Pritchard, E.E.
1937 Witchcraft, Oracles and Magic among the Azande. Oxford: The Clarendon Press.

Filliozat, Jean
1964 The Classical Doctrine of Indian Medicine: Its Origins and Its Greek Parallels. Translated by Dev Raj Chanana. Delhi: Munshiram Manoharlal.

Filmer, Paul
1972 On Harold Garfinkel's Ethnomethodology. In New Directions in Sociological Theory. Paul Filmer et al., eds. Pp. 203-34. Cambridge: M.I.T. Press.

Foucault, Michel
1965 Madness and Civilization: A History of Insanity in the Age of Reason. Translated by Richard Howard. New York: Pantheon Books.

Freed, Stanley A. and Ruth S. Freed
1964 Spirit possession as illness in a North Indian village. Ethnology 3:152-71.

Garfinkel, Harold
1967 Studies in Ethnomethodology. Englewood Cliffs, NJ: Prentice Hall.

Geertz, Clifford
1975 Common sense as a cultural system. The Antioch Review 33:5-26.

Giorgi, Amedeo
1970 Psychology as a Human Science: A Phenomenologically Based Approach. New York: Harper and Row.

Glaser, Barney G. and Anselm L. Strauss
1967 The Discovery of Grounded Theory. Chicago: Aldine Publishing Company.

Gluckman, Max, ed.
1972 The Allocation of Responsibility. Manchester: Manchester University Press.

Gould, Harold A.
1957 The implications of technological change for folk and scientific medicine. American Anthropologist 59:507-16.

1965 Modern medicine and folk cognition in rural India. Human Organization 24:201-8.

Goyeche, R.
1972 Yoga as psychotherapy. Journal of the Yoga Institute 18(1):4-7.

Gupta, Brahmananda
1976 Indigenous medicine in nineteenth and twentieth century Bengal. In Asian Medical Systems: A Comparative Study. Charles Leslie, ed. Pp. 368-82. Berkeley: University of California Press.

Gupta, Nitya N.
1956 Influence of Hindu culture and social symptoms on psychosomatic disease in India. Psychosomatic Medicine 18:506-10.

Harper, Edward B.
1957 Shamanism in South India. Southwestern Journal of Anthropology 13:267-87.

Harper, Edward B.
1963 Spirit possession and social structure. In Anthropology on the March: Recent Studies of Indian Beliefs, Attitudes, and Social Institutions. L.K. Bala Ratnam, ed. Pp. 165-97. Madras: The Book Centre.

Hasan, Khwaja A.
1967 The Cultural Frontier of Health in Village India: Case Study of a North Indian Village. Bombay: Manaktalas.

Horton, Robin
1967a African traditional thought and Western science; Part I: From tradition to science. Africa 37:50-52.

1967b African traditional thought and Western science; Part II: The 'closed' and 'open' predicaments. Africa 37:155-87.

Inden, Ronald B.
1976 Marriage and Rank in Bengal: A History of Caste and Clan in Middle Period Bengal. Berkeley: University of California Press.

Inden, Ronald B. and Ralph W. Nicholas
1977 Kinship in Bengali Culture. Chicago: University of Chicago Press.

Jacobs, Hans
1961 Western Psychotherapy and Hindu Sadhana: A Contribution to Comparative Studies in Psychology and Metaphysics. London: Allen & Unwin.

Jaggi, O.P.
1973a History of Science and Technology in India, Vol. III: Folk Medicine. Delhi: Atma Ram & Sons.

1973b History of Science and Technology in India, Vol. IV: Indian System of Medicine. Delhi: Atma Ram & Sons.

Janzen, John M.
1978 The Quest for Therapy in Lower Zaire. Berkeley: University of California Press.

Joint Commission on Mental Illness and Health
1961 Action for Mental Health: Final Report. New York: Basic Books.

Jolly, Julius
1951 Indian Medicine. Translated by C.G. Kashikar. Poona: C.G. Kashikar.

Joshi, H.M.
1964 Indian approach to psychology. Darshana International 4(2):58-69.

Kakar, D.N.
1972 The health centre doctor and spirit medium in a North Indian village. Eastern Anthropologist 25:249-58.

Kakar, Sudhir
1968 The human life cycle: the traditional Hindu view and the psychology of Erik Erikson. Philosophy East and West 28:127-36.

1978 The Inner World: A Psychoanalytic Study of Childhood and Society in India. Delhi: Oxford University Press.

Kapur, R.L.
1979 The role of traditional healers in mental health care in rural India. Social Science and Medicine 13B:27-31.

Khare, R.S.
1963 Folk medicine and a North Indian village. Human Organization 22:36-40.

Kleinman, Arthur
1980 Patients and Healers in the Context of Culture: An Exploration of the Borderland between Anthropology, Medicine, and Psychiatry. Berkeley: University of California Press.

Kleinman, Arthur, et al., eds.
1978 Culture and Healing in Asian Societies: Anthropological, Psychiatric, and Public Health Studies. Cambridge, MA: Schenkman Publishing Company.

Kunstadter, Peter
1978 Do cultural differences make any difference? Choice points in medical systems available in northwestern Thailand. In Culture and Healing in Asian Societies. Arthur Kleinman et al., eds. Pp. 185-218. Cambridge, MA: Schenkman Publishing Company.

Kutumbiah, P.
1962 Ancient Indian Medicine. Bombay: Orient Longmans Ltd.

Labov, William and David Fanshel
1977 Therapeutic Discourse: Psychotherapy as Conversation. New York: Academic Press.

Leach, Edmund
1970 Levi-Strauss. London: William Collins & Co.

Leslie, Charles
1967 Professional and popular health cultures in South Asia: needed research in medical sociology and anthropology. In Understanding Science and Technology in India and Pakistan. Ward Morehouse, ed. Pp. 27-42. New York: Occasional Publications, No. 8, Foreign Area Materials Center, State University of New York.

1973 The professionalizing ideology of medical revivalism. In Entrepreneurship and Modernization of Occupational Cultures in South Asia. Milton Singer, ed. Pp. 216-42. Durham: Duke University Press.

1974 The modernization of Asian medical systems. In Rethinking Modernization: Anthropological Perspectives. John J. Poggie, Jr. and Robert N. Lynch, eds. Pp. 69-108. Westport, CT: Greenwood Press.

1976a Asian Medical Systems: A Comparative Study. Berkeley: University of California Press.

1976b The ambiguities of medical revivalism in modern India. In Asian Medical Systems: A Comparative Study. Charles Leslie, ed. Pp. 356-67. Berkeley: University of California Press.

Leslie, Charles
1978 Pluralism and integration in the Indian and Chinese medical systems. In Culture and Healing in Asian Societies: Anthropological, Psychiatric, and Public Health Studies. Arthur Kleinman et al., eds. Pp. 235-52. Cambridge, MA: Schenkman Publishing Company.

1980 Medical pluralism in world perspective. Social Science and Medicine 14B:191-95.

Lyons, John
1970 Noam Chomsky. New York: Viking Press.

Manning, Peter K. and Horatio Fabrega, Jr.
1973 The experience of self and body: health and illness in the Chiapas highlands. In Phenomenological Sociology: Issues and Applications. George Psathas, ed. Pp. 251-301. New York: John Wiley and Sons.

Marriott, McKim
1955 Western medicine in a village of northern India. In Health, Culture, and Community: Case Studies of Public Reactions to Health Programs. Benjamin D. Paul, ed. Pp. 239-68. New York: Russell Sage Foundation.

1976 Hindu transactions: Diversity without dualism. In Transaction and Meaning: Directions in the Anthropology of Exchange and Symbolic Behavior. Bruce Kapferer, ed. Pp. 109-42. Philadelphia: Institute for the Study of Human Issues.

Marriott, McKim and Ronald B. Inden
1976 Toward an ethnosociology of South Asian caste systems. In The New Wind: Changing Identities in South Asia. Kenneth David, ed. Pp. 227-38. The Hague: Mouton.

Masson, J. Moussaieff
1974 Sex and yoga: psychoanalysis and the Indian religious experience. Journal of Indian Philosophy 2:307-20.

Mehan, Hugh
1978 Structuring school structure. Harvard Educational Review 48:32-64.

Mills, C. Wright
1940 Situated actions and vocabularies of motive. American Sociological Review 5:904-13.

Murphy, Gardner and Lois B. Murphy, eds.
1968 Asian Psychology. New York: Basic Books.

Nicholas, Ralph W. and Aditi Nath Sarkar
1976 The Fever Demon and Census Commissioner: Sitala mythology in eighteenth- and nineteenth-century Bengal. In Bengal: Studies in Literature, Society and History. Marvin Davis, ed. Pp. 3-68. East Lansing: Michigan State University, Asian Studies Center South Asian Series, Occasional Paper No. 27.

Obeyesekere, Gananath
1976 The impact of Ayurvedic ideas on the culture and individual in Sri Lanka. In Asian Medical Systems: A Comparative Study. Charles Leslie, ed. Pp. 201-26. Berkeley: University of California Press.

Opler, Morris E.
1958 Spirit possession in a rural area of northern India. In Reader in Comparative Religion. William A. Lessa and Evon Z. Vogt, eds. Pp. 553-66. New York: Harper and Row.

1963 The cultural definition of illness in village India. Human Organization 22:32-35.

Pal, Kumar
1971 Comparison of yoga and psychoanalysis. Darshana International 11(1):49-67.

Phillipson, Michael
1972 Theory, methodology and conceptualization. In New Directions in Sociological Theory. Paul Filmer, et al., eds. Pp. 77-116. Cambridge: MIT Press.

Pike, K.
1954 Emic and etic standpoints for the description of behavior. In Language in Relation to a Unified Theory of the Structure of Human Behavior. K. Pike, ed. Pp. 8-28. Glendale, CA: Summer Institute of Linguistics.

Ramana, C.V.
1964 On the early history and development of psychoanalysis in India. American Psychoanalytic Association Journal 12:110-34.

Rao, S.K. Ramachandra
1962 Development of Psychological Thought in India. Mysore: Kavyalaya Publishers.

Rastogi, V.S. et al.
1976 Somatic symptoms in neurosis: a cross-cultural study. Indian Journal of Psychiatry 18:103-8.

Rubington, Earl and Martin S. Weinberg
1978 Deviance: The Interactionist Perspective. Third edition. New York: McMillan Publishing Company.

Sacks, Harvey
1972 An initial investigation of the usability of conversational data for doing sociology. In Studies in Social Interaction. David Sudnow, ed. Pp. 31-74. New York: Free Press.

1974 On the analyzability of stories by children. In Ethnomethodology. Roy Turner, ed. Pp. 216-32. Baltimore: Penguin Books.

Schegloff, Emmanuel and Harvey Sacks
1973 Opening up closings. Semiotica 8:289-327.

Schur, Edwin M.
1971 Labeling Deviant Behavior: Its Sociological Implications. New York: Harper and Row.

Schutz, Alfred
1970 Alfred Schutz on Phenomenology and Social Relations. Helmut R. Wagner, ed. Chicago: University of Chicago Press.

Scott, Marvin B. and Stanford M. Lyman
1968 Accounts. American Sociological Review 33:46-62.

Sharma, P.V.
1972 Indian Medicine in the Classical Age. Chowkhamba Sanskrit Series, Vol. 85. Varanasi: Chowkhamba Sanskrit Series Office.

Smith, Dorothy
1974 Theorizing as ideology. In Ethnomethodology. Roy Turner, ed. Pp. 41-44. Baltimore: Penguin Books.

Somasundaram, O.
1973 Religious treatment of mental illness in Tamil Nadu. Indian Journal of Psychiatry 15(1):38-48.

Sperber, Dan
1974 Rethinking Symbolism. Cambridge: Cambridge University Press.

Spradley, James P., ed.
1972 Culture and Cognition: Rules, Maps and Plans. San Francisco: Chandler Publishing Company.

Spratt, Philip
1966 Hindu Culture and Personality: A Psychoanalytic Study. Bombay: Manaktalas.

Srinavasa, D.K. and S. Trivedi
1982 Knowledge and attitude of mental diseases in a rural community of South India. Social Science and Medicine 16:1635-39.

Sturtevant, William C.
1964 Studies in Ethnoscience. American Anthropologist 66:99-131.

Surya, N.C.
1969 Ego structure in the Hindu joint family: some considerations. In Mental Health Research in Asia and the Pacific. William Caudill and Tsung-yi Lin, eds. Pp. 381-92. Honolulu: East-West Center Press.

Szasz, Thomas S.
1970 Ideology and Insanity: Essays on the Psychiatric Dehumanization of Man. Garden City, NY: Anchor Books.

1974 The Myth of Mental Illness: Foundations of a Theory of Personal Conduct. New York: Harper and Row Publishers.

Turner, Roy
1974 Words, utterances, and activities. In Ethnomethodology. Roy Turner, ed. Pp. 197-215. Baltimore: Penguin Books.

Turner, Victor W.
1964 A Ndembu doctor in practice. In Magic, Faith, and Healing: Studies in Primitive Psychiatry Today. Ari Kiev, ed. Pp. 230-63. New York: Free Press.

Turner, Victor W.
1967 The Forest of Symbols: Aspects of Ndembu Ritual. Ithaca: Cornell University Press.

Vahia, N.S.
1969 A therapy based upon some concepts prevalent in India. Indian Journal of Psychiatry 11(1 and 2):7-14.

Vahia, N.S. et al.
1966 Some ancient Indian concepts in the treatment of psychiatric disorders. British Journal of Psychiatry 112:1089-96.

1972 A deconditioning therapy based upon concepts of Patanjali. International Journal of Social Psychiatry 18:61-68.

1973a Further experience with the therapy based upon concepts of Patanjali in the treatment of psychiatric disorders. Indian Journal of Psychiatry 15:32-37.

1973b Psychophysiologic therapy based upon the concepts of Patanjali. American Journal of Psychotherapy 27:557-65.

Wadley, Susan Snow
1975 Shakti: Power in the Conceptual Structure of Karimpur Religion. University of Chicago Studies in Anthropology, Series in Social, Cultural, and Linguistic Anthropology, No. 2. Chicago: Department of Anthropology, University of Chicago.

Weider, D. Lawrence
1974 Telling the code. In Ethnomethodology. Roy Turner, ed. Pp. 144-72. Baltimore: Penguin Books.

Weiss, Mitchell
1975 Psychopathology in classical India. Unpublished.

1976 Psychopathology in early Ayurvedic texts. Paper presented at the 186th Annual Meeting of the American Oriental Society, Philadelphia, PA.

Young, Allan
1976 Some implications of medical beliefs and practices for social anthropology. American Anthropologist 78:5-24.

Zimmer, Heinrich R.
1948 Hindu Medicine. Baltimore: Johns Hopkins University Press.

Zimmerman, Don H.
1974 Fact as a practical accomplishment. In Ethnomethodology. Roy Turner, ed. Pp. 128-43. Baltimore: Penguin Books.

Zimmerman, Don H. and Melvin Pollner
1970 The everyday world as a phenomenon. In Understanding Everyday Life: Toward the Reconstruction of Sociological Knowledge. Jack D. Douglas, ed. Pp. 80-104. Chicago: Aldine Publishing Company.

INDEX

Notes: n refers to footnotes. Titles are italicized. Words in a language other than English are underlined.

ABOUT THE AUTHOR

Deborah P. Bhattacharyya first went to India in 1963 at age 19. As a volunteer in Service Civil International, she worked in several village projects in India and Sri Lanka. Returning to school, she received her B.A. and M.A. from Southern Illinois University and the Ph.D. from Indiana University. Dr. Bhattacharyya is currently an Assistant Professor at DePauw University, where she teaches courses in social work and social psychology as well as South Asian culture and society. Her most recent project is an off-campus study program, Asian Odyssey, through which undergraduates visit India and China.